A Colour Atlas of Head and Neck Anatomy

Copyright © R.M.H. McMinn, R.T. Hutchings, B.M. Logan, 1981
Published by Wolfe Medical Publications Ltd, 1981
Printed by Royal Smeets Offset b.v., Weert, Netherlands
ISBN 0 7234 0755 X
6th impression, 1990

A CIP catalogue record for this book is available from the British
Library.

This book is one of the titles in the series of Wolfe Medical Atlases,
a series that brings together the world's largest systematic published
collection of diagnostic colour photographs.

For a full list of Atlases in the series, plus forthcoming titles and
details of our surgical, dental and veterinary Atlases, please write to
Wolfe Medical Publications Ltd, 2–16 Torrington Place, London
WC1E 7LT, England.

A Colour Atlas of

Head and Neck Anatomy

R M H McMinn

Emeritus Professor of Anatomy,
Royal College of Surgeons of England
and University of London

R T Hutchings

Photographer
Formerly Chief Medical Laboratory
Scientific Officer, Royal College
of Surgeons of England

B M Logan

Prosector
Department of Anatomy
Royal College of Surgeons of England

Wolfe Medical Publications Ltd

To
Christopher and Jacqueline
Sam and Isabel
and Evelyn

Preface

The reception given to 'A Colour Atlas of Human Anatomy', which dealt with the whole body, has encouraged us to produce a companion volume dealing specifically with the head and neck, in order to meet the anatomical needs of those who are concerned particularly with this region of the body. This book is not a reprint of relevant head and neck sections of the earlier atlas; it is a completely new work, with new specimens and new illustrations. The same format has been retained, namely natural size colour photographs with identification numbers overlying individual structures and an adjacent key, as this has proved to be universally popular with both undergraduates and postgraduates. This system allows students to test their own knowledge by covering up the key. The notes that accompany the identification keys help to emphasise certain important points, but there has been no attempt to give a complete commentary on everything illustrated. The book is essentially an atlas designed to complement existing texts, dissecting manuals and other atlases, not to replace them.

We hope that our contribution will assist in the understanding of an intricate but fascinating part of the body, and that the quality of presentation will make even study for examinations a pleasurable experience.

R.M.H. McMinn
R.T. Hutchings
B.M. Logan

Acknowledgements

We are much indebted to our colleague Dr D.H. Bosman for placing his eagle eye and expert anatomical knowledge at our disposal. We are also grateful to Professor T.W. Glenister and Messrs Adam, Rouilly for the loan of osteological material, to Dr Oscar Craig for radiological advice, to Sue and Maggie, to Steve Logan, and to Gina Howes for the typing and retyping of the manuscript.

The illustrations of museum specimens are reproduced by courtesy of the President of the Royal College of Surgeons of England, to whom we also express our thanks.

Contents

The Skull

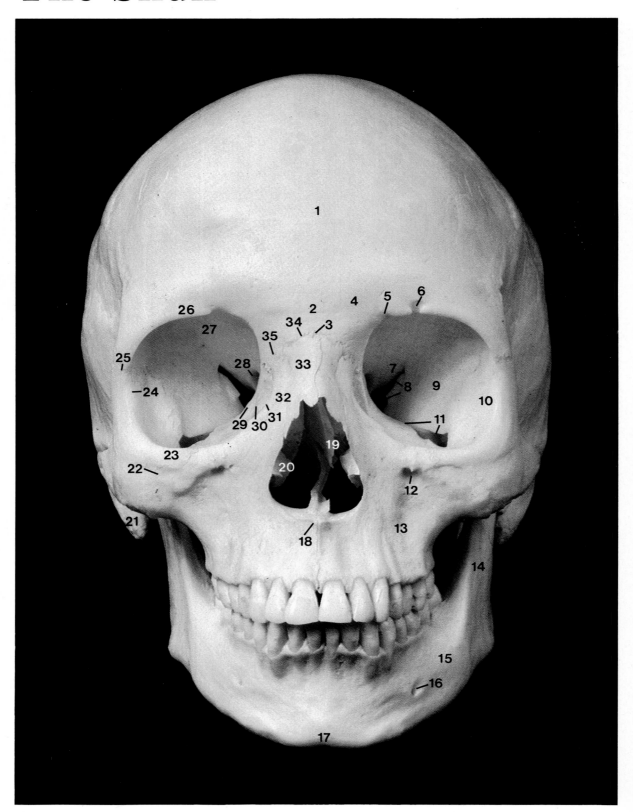

THE SKULL

From the front

1 Frontal bone
2 Glabella
3 Nasion
4 Superciliary arch
5 Frontal notch
6 Supra-orbital foramen
7 Lesser wing of sphenoid bone
8 Superior orbital fissure
9 Greater wing of sphenoid bone
10 Zygomatic bone
11 Inferior orbital fissure
12 Infra-orbital foramen
13 Maxilla
14 Ramus ⎫
15 Body ⎪
16 Mental foramen ⎬ of mandible
17 Mental protuberance ⎪
18 Anterior nasal spine ⎭
19 Nasal septum
20 Inferior nasal concha
21 Mastoid process
22 Zygomaticomaxillary suture
23 Infra-orbital margin
24 Marginal tubercle
25 Frontozygomatic suture
26 Supra-orbital margin
27 Orbital part of frontal bone
28 Optic canal
29 Posterior lacrimal crest
30 Fossa for lacrimal sac
31 Anterior lacrimal crest
32 Frontal process of maxilla
33 Nasal bone
34 Frontonasal suture
35 Frontomaxillary suture

● The term skull includes the mandible; the cranium is the skull without the mandible, but these definitions are not always strictly observed.

● The calvaria (a term not often used) is the upper part of the skull that encloses the brain (i.e. the cranial cavity) and has a roof or skull cap, and a floor known as the base of the skull.

● The anterior part of the skull forms the facial skeleton.

● The cavities of the skull:
Cranial cavity, containing the brain and its membranes.
Nasal cavity, divided by the midline nasal septum into right and left halves.
Orbits or orbital cavities, right and left, in which the eyeballs are lodged.

● The bones of the skull:

Unpaired	Paired
Frontal	Maxilla
Ethmoid	Nasal
Sphenoid	Lacrimal
Vomer	Inferior nasal concha
Occipital	Palatine
Mandible	Zygomatic
	Temporal
	Parietal

● Important landmarks on the outside of the skull include:
the orbits
the anterior nasal aperture (piriform aperture)
the zygomatic arch
pterion
the external acoustic meatus
the hard palate
the posterior nasal apertures (choanae)
the foramen magnum
the mastoid process
the styloid process

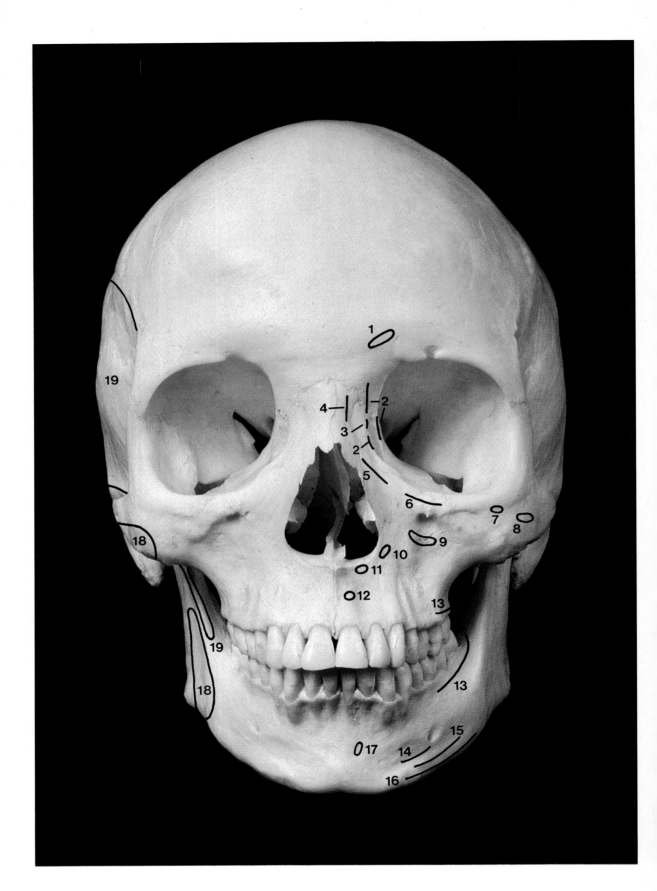

THE SKULL

From the front. Muscle attachments

1 Corrugator supercilii
2 Orbicularis oculi
3 Medial palpebral ligament
4 Procerus
5 Levator labii superioris alaeque nasi
6 Levator labii superioris
7 Zygomaticus minor
8 Zygomaticus major
9 Levator anguli oris
10 Nasalis (transverse part)
11 Nasalis (alar part)
12 Depressor septi
13 Buccinator
14 Depressor labii inferioris
15 Depressor anguli oris
16 Platysma
17 Mentalis
18 Masseter
19 Temporalis

● The supra-orbital, infra-orbital and mental foramina lie approximately in the same vertical plane.

● The infra-orbital foramen is 0.5 cm below the infra-orbital margin, immediately below the pupil (with the eye looking forwards) and in the long axis of the second premolar tooth.

● The attachment of levator labii superioris is *above* the infra-orbital foramen, and the attachment of levator anguli oris *below* the foramen.

● The mental foramen lies below and between the apices of the two premolar teeth.

● The attachment of depressor labii inferioris lies *in front* of the mental foramen and the attachment of depressor anguli oris *below* the foramen.

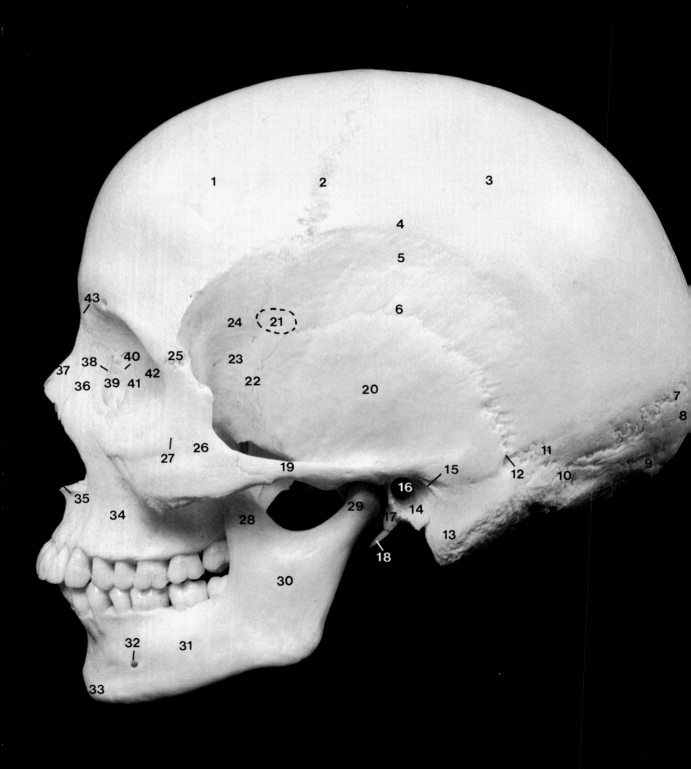

THE SKULL

From the left

1 Frontal bone
2 Coronal suture
3 Parietal bone
4 Superior ⎫
5 Inferior ⎬ temporal line
6 Squamosal suture
7 Lambdoid suture
8 Occipital bone
9 External occipital protuberance
10 Occipitomastoid suture
11 Parietomastoid suture
12 Asterion
13 Mastoid process
14 Tympanic part of temporal bone
15 Suprameatal triangle
16 External acoustic meatus
17 Sheath of styloid process
18 Styloid process
19 Zygomatic arch
20 Squamous part of temporal bone
21 Pterion
22 Sphenosquamosal suture
23 Greater wing of sphenoid bone
24 Sphenofrontal suture
25 Frontozygomatic suture
26 Zygomatic bone
27 Zygomaticofacial foramen
28 Coronoid process ⎫
29 Condylar process ⎪
30 Ramus ⎪
31 Body ⎬ of mandible
32 Mental foramen ⎪
33 Mental protuberance ⎭
34 Maxilla
35 Anterior nasal spine
36 Frontal process of maxilla
37 Nasal bone
38 Anterior lacrimal crest
39 Fossa for lacrimal sac
40 Posterior lacrimal crest
41 Lacrimal bone
42 Orbital part of ethmoid bone
43 Nasion

● Some anatomical points of the skull:

Nasion: the point of articulation between the two nasal bones and the frontal bone.

Inion: the central point of the external occipital protuberance (which is *not* the most posterior part of the occipital bone).

Bregma: at the junction of the sagittal and coronal sutures (i.e. between the frontal and the two parietal bones). In the newborn skull the anterior fontanelle is in this region.

Lambda: at the junction of the sagittal and lambdoid sutures (i.e. between the occipital and the two parietal bones). In the newborn skull the posterior fontanelle is in this region.

Pterion: an H-shaped area (not a single point) where the frontal, parietal, squamous part of the temporal and greater wing of the sphenoid bones articulate. It is an important landmark on the side of the skull as it overlies the anterior branch of the middle meningeal artery. In the newborn skull the sphenoidal fontanelle is in this region.

Asterion: at the junction of the lambdoid, parietomastoid and occipitomastoid sutures (i.e. between the occipital, parietal and temporal bones). In the newborn skull the mastoid fontanelle is in this region.

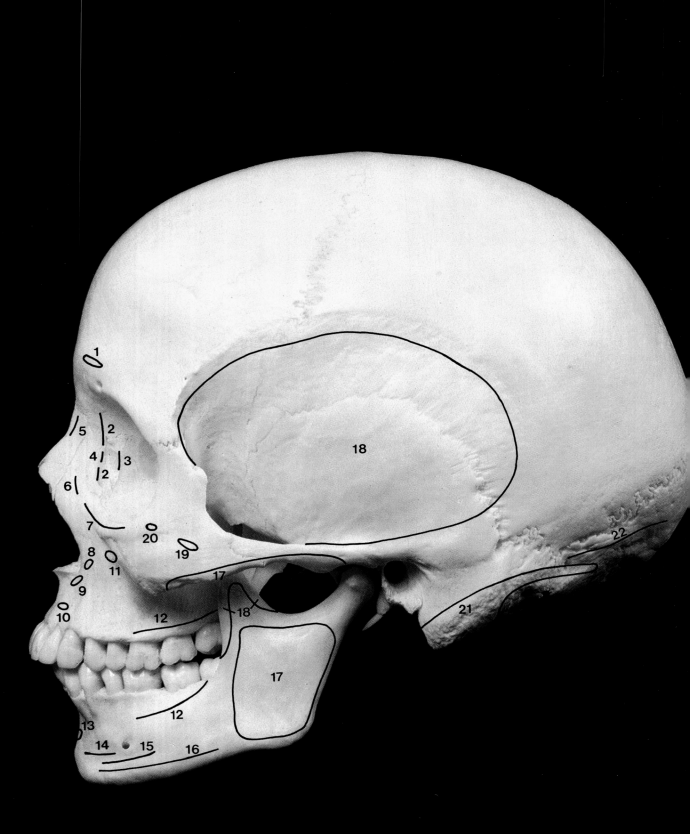

THE SKULL

From the left. Muscle attachments

1 Corrugator supercilii
2 Orbicularis oculi (orbital and palpebral parts)
3 Orbicularis oculi (lacrimal part)
4 Medial palpebral ligament
5 Procerus
6 Levator labii superioris alaeque nasi
7 Levator labii superioris
8 Nasalis (transverse part)
9 Nasalis (alar part)
10 Depressor septi
11 Levator anguli oris
12 Buccinator
13 Mentalis
14 Depressor labii inferioris
15 Depressor anguli oris
16 Platysma
17 Masseter
18 Temporalis
19 Zygomaticus major
20 Zygomaticus minor
21 Sternocleidomastoid
22 Occipital belly of occipitofrontalis

● The buccinator has a bony attachment to the upper and lower jaws opposite the three molar teeth.

● The medial palpebral ligament and the orbital and palpebral parts of orbicularis oculi are attached to the *anterior* lacrimal crest; the lacrimal part of orbicularis oculi is attached to the *posterior* lacrimal crest.

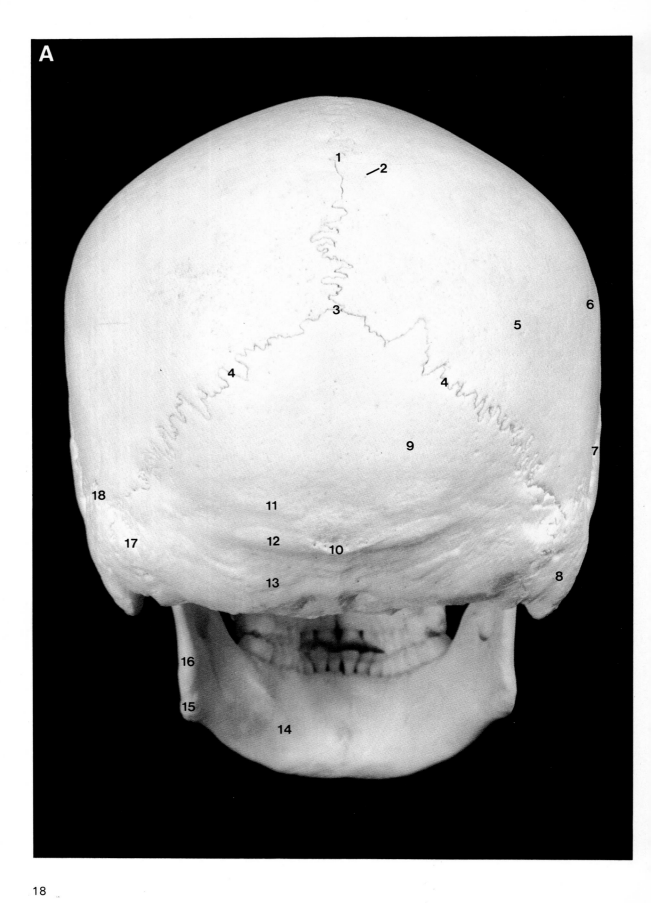

THE SKULL

A From behind
B From behind, with sutural bones

 1 Sagittal suture
 2 Parietal foramen
 3 Lambda
 4 Lambdoid suture
 5 Parietal bone
 6 Parietal tuberosity
 7 Temporal bone
 8 Mastoid process
 9 Squamous part of occipital bone
10 External occipital protuberance (inion)
11 Supreme ⎤
12 Superior ⎬ nuchal line
13 Inferior ⎦
14 Body ⎤
15 Angle ⎬ of mandible
16 Ramus ⎦
17 Occipitomastoid suture
18 Parietomastoid suture
19 Sutural bones

● Sutural bones arise from separate centres of ossification that may occur within cranial sutures. They are commonest in the lambdoid suture and have no significance.

● In this skull there has been bony fusion in some sutural areas.

● The vertex of the skull is the highest point; it is on the sagittal suture a few centimetres behind bregma (see page 20).

● The occiput is the most posterior part of the skull; it is on the midline of the occipital bone a few centimetres above the external occipital protuberance.

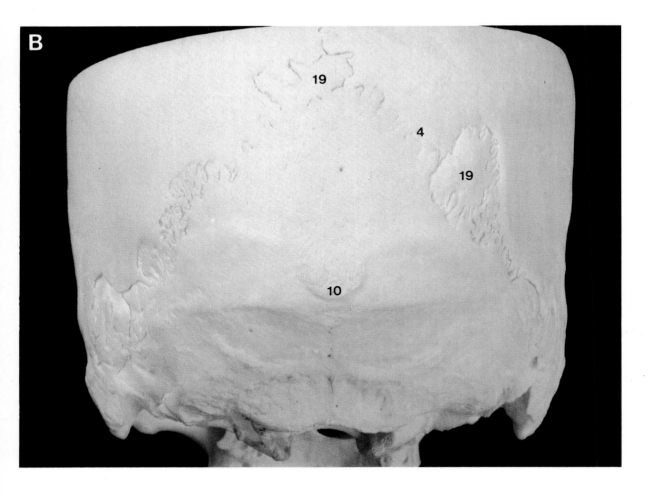

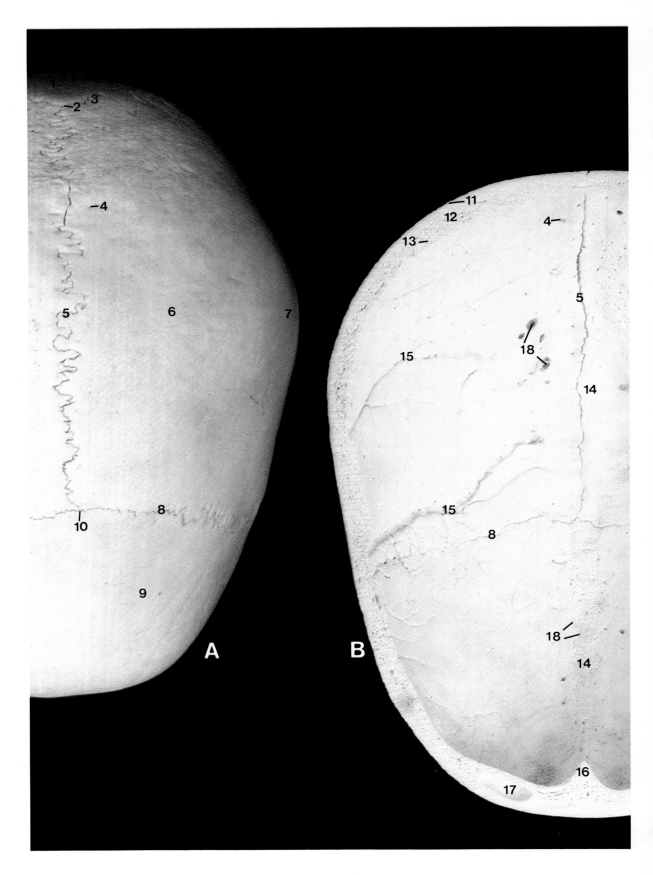

THE SKULL

The cranial vault

A External surface (left half)
B Internal surface (left half)

1 Occipital bone
2 Lambda
3 Lambdoid suture
4 Parietal foramen
5 Sagittal suture
6 Parietal bone
7 Parietal tuberosity
8 Coronal suture
9 Frontal bone
10 Bregma
11 Outer table ⎫
12 Diploë ⎬ of parietal bone
13 Inner table ⎭
14 Groove for superior sagittal sinus
15 Grooves for middle meningeal vessels
16 Frontal crest
17 Frontal sinus
18 Depressions for arachnoid granulations

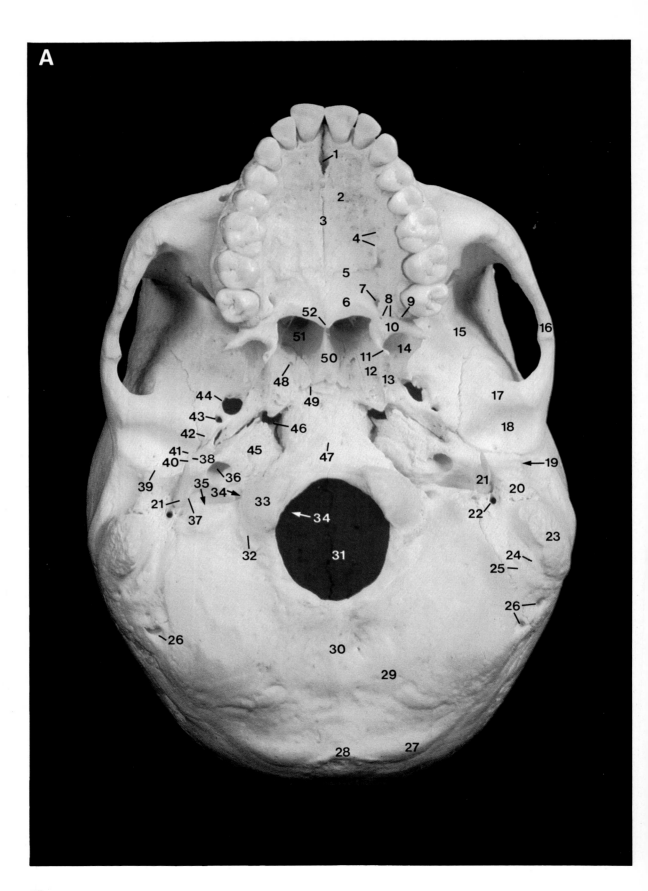

THE SKULL

The external surface of the base

A From below
B From below and behind

1 Incisive fossa	31 Foramen magnum
2 Palatine process of maxilla	32 Condylar canal
3 Median palatine suture	33 Occipital condyle
4 Palatine grooves and spines	34 Hypoglossal canal
5 Transverse palatine suture	35 Jugular foramen
6 Horizontal plate of palatine bone	36 Carotid canal
7 Greater palatine foramen	37 Sheath of styloid process
8 Lesser palatine foramina	38 Petrotympanic fissure
9 Tuberosity of maxilla	39 Squamotympanic fissure
10 Pyramidal process of palatine bone	40 Tegmen tympani
11 Pterygoid hamulus	41 Petrosquamous fissure
12 Medial pterygoid plate	42 Spine of sphenoid bone
13 Scaphoid fossa	43 Foramen spinosum
14 Lateral pterygoid plate	44 Foramen ovale
15 Infratemporal crest	45 Apex of petrous part of temporal bone
16 Zygomatic arch	46 Foramen lacerum
17 Articular tubercle	47 Pharyngeal tubercle
18 Mandibular fossa	48 Palatovaginal canal
19 External acoustic meatus	49 Vomerovaginal canal
20 Tympanic part of temporal bone	50 Vomer
21 Styloid process	51 Posterior nasal aperture (choana)
22 Stylomastoid foramen	52 Posterior nasal spine
23 Mastoid process	53 Infratemporal surface } of maxilla
24 Mastoid notch	54 Zygomatic process }
25 Occipital groove	55 Zygomaticomaxillary suture
26 Mastoid foramen (double on left)	56 Zygomaticotemporal foramen
27 Superior nuchal line	57 Inferior orbital fissure
28 External occipital protuberance	58 Inferior
29 Inferior nuchal line	59 Middle } nasal concha
30 External occipital crest	60 Superior

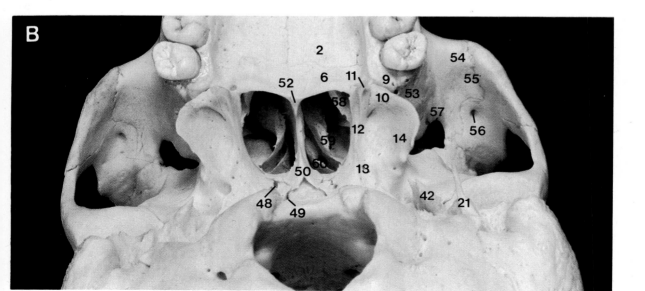

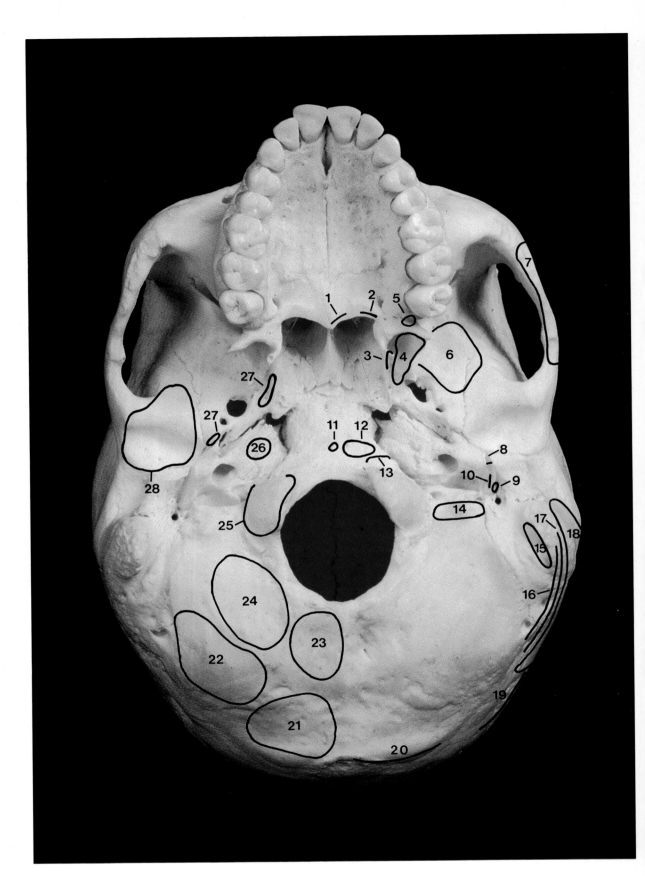

THE SKULL

The external surface of the base.
Muscle attachments

1 Musculus uvulae
2 Palatopharyngeus
3 Superior constrictor of pharynx
4 Medial pterygoid (deep head)
5 Medial pterygoid (superficial head)
6 Lateral pterygoid (upper head)
7 Masseter
8 Styloglossus
9 Stylohyoid
10 Stylopharyngeus
11 Pharyngeal raphe
12 Longus capitus
13 Rectus capitis anterior
14 Rectus capitis lateralis
15 Posterior belly of digastric
16 Longissimus capitis
17 Splenius capitis
18 Sternocleidomastoid
19 Occipital belly of occipitofrontalis
20 Trapezius
21 Semispinalis capitis
22 Superior oblique
23 Rectus capitis posterior minor
24 Rectus capitis posterior major
25 Capsule of atlanto-occipital joint
26 Levator veli palatini
27 Tensor veli palatini
28 Capsule of temporomandibular joint

● Principal skull foramina and their contents:
(for more precise details see pages 223–225)

Supra-orbital foramen
    Supra-orbital nerve and vessels
Infra-orbital foramen
    Infra-orbital nerve and vessels
Mental foramen
    Mental nerve and vessels
Mandibular foramen
    Inferior alveolar nerve and vessels
Optic canal
    Optic nerve
    Ophthalmic artery
Superior orbital fissure
    Ophthalmic nerve and veins
    Oculomotor, trochlear and abducent nerves
Inferior orbital fissure
    Maxillary nerve
Sphenopalatine foramen
    Sphenopalatine artery
    Nasal branches of pterygopalatine ganglion
Foramen rotundum
    Maxillary nerve
Foramen ovale
    Mandibular and lesser petrosal nerves
Foramen spinosum
    Middle meningeal vessels
Foramen lacerum
    Internal carotid artery (entering from behind and emerging above)
    Greater petrosal nerve (entering from behind and leaving anteriorly as the nerve of the pterygoid canal)
Carotid canal
    Internal carotid artery and nerve
Jugular foramen
    Inferior petrosal sinus
    Glossopharyngeal, vagus and accessory nerves
    Internal jugular vein (emerging below)
Internal acoustic meatus
    Facial and vestibulocochlear nerves
    Labyrinthine artery
Hypoglossal canal
    Hypoglossal nerve
Stylomastoid foramen
    Facial nerve
Foramen magnum
    Medulla oblongata and meninges
    Vertebral and anterior and posterior spinal arteries
    Accessory nerves

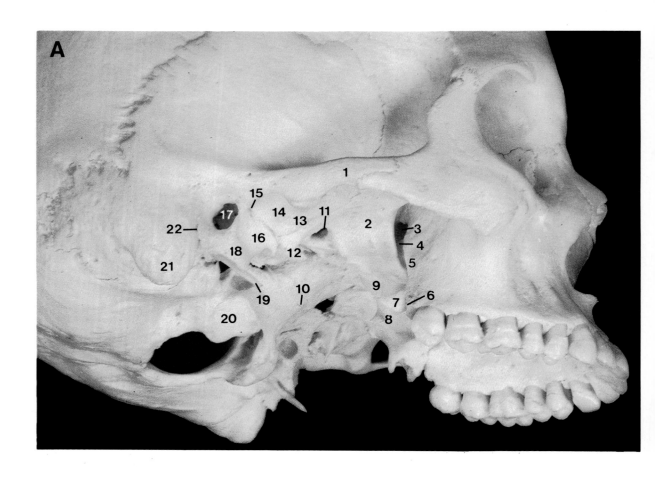

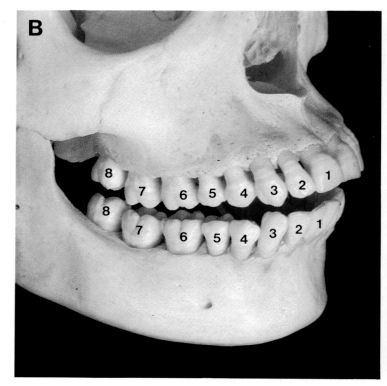

THE SKULL

A The right infratemporal region, obliquely from below

1 Zygomatic arch
2 Lateral pterygoid plate
3 Sphenopalatine foramen
4 Pterygomaxillary fissure
5 Infratemporal surface of maxilla
6 Tuberosity of maxilla
7 Pyramidal process of palatine bone
8 Pterygoid hamulus
9 Medial pterygoid plate
10 Pharyngeal tubercle
11 Foramen ovale
12 Spine of sphenoid bone
13 Articular tubercle
14 Mandibular fossa
15 Squamotympanic fissure
16 Tympanic part of temporal bone
17 External acoustic meatus
18 Sheath of styloid process
19 Styloid process
20 Occipital condyle
21 Mastoid process
22 Tympanomastoid fissure

B Permanent dentition. The teeth of the upper and lower jaws in the adult, from the right and in front

1 Central ⎫
2 Lateral ⎬ incisor
3 Canine
4 First ⎫
5 Second ⎬ premolar
6 First ⎫
7 Second ⎬ molar
8 Third

● The corresponding teeth of the upper and lower jaws have corresponding names. In clinical dentistry the teeth are often identified by the numbers 1 to 8 as listed here, rather than by name. Thus, 'right upper 6' refers to the right upper first molar tooth.

● The third molar tooth is sometimes called the wisdom tooth.

● In the deciduous dentition of the child ('milk teeth'), there are central and lateral incisors and canines in corresponding positions to the permanent teeth of the same name, and first and second deciduous molars in the positions of the permanent premolars.

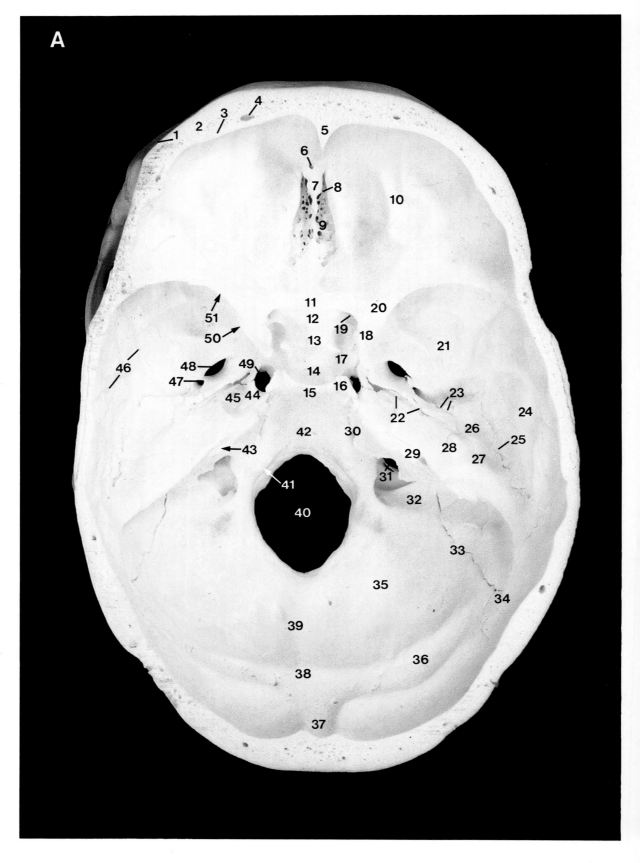

THE SKULL

The internal surface of the base. The anterior, middle and posterior cranial fossae

A From above
B Part of the middle cranial fossa, from above, right and behind
C Left part of the middle cranial fossa, from above, showing the occasional foramina

1 Outer table
2 Diploë
3 Inner table
4 Frontal sinus (upper extremity)
5 Frontal crest
6 Foramen caecum
7 Crista galli
8 Groove for anterior ethmoidal nerve and vessels
9 Cribriform plate of ethmoid bone
10 Orbital part of frontal bone
11 Jugum of sphenoid bone
12 Prechiasmatic groove
13 Tuberculum sellae
14 Pituitary fossa (sella turcica)
15 Dorsum sellae
16 Posterior clinoid process
17 Carotid groove
18 Anterior clinoid process
19 Optic canal
20 Lesser wing of sphenoid bone
21 Greater wing of sphenoid bone
22 Hiatus and groove for greater petrosal nerve
23 Hiatus and groove for lesser petrosal nerve
24 Squamous part of temporal bone
25 Petrosquamous fissure
26 Tegmen tympani
27 Arcuate eminence
28 Petrous part of temporal bone
29 Groove for superior petrosal sinus
30 Groove for inferior petrosal sinus and petro-occipital suture
31 Jugular foramen
32 Groove for sigmoid sinus
33 Occipitomastoid suture
34 Mastoid (postero-inferior) angle of parietal bone

35 Occipital bone
36 Groove for transverse sinus
37 Groove for superior sagittal sinus
38 Internal occipital protuberance
39 Internal occipital crest
40 Foramen magnum
41 Hypoglossal canal
42 Clivus
43 Internal acoustic meatus
44 Apex of petrous part of temporal bone
45 Trigeminal impression
46 Grooves for middle meningeal vessels
47 Foramen spinosum
48 Foramen ovale
49 Foramen lacerum
50 Foramen rotundum
51 Superior orbital fissure
52 Venous (emissary sphenoidal) foramen (of Vesalius)
53 Petrosal (innominate) foramen

● For details of the bones of the cranial fossae see pages 64–67.
● The foramina rotundum, ovale and spinosum are always present within the greater wing of the sphenoid bone; the venous (emissary sphenoidal) foramen (of Vesalius) and the petrosal (innominate) foramen are occasional additions (as in C).
● The openings in the anterior cranial fossa are:
the foramen caecum
the foramina of the cribriform plate of the ethmoid bone
● The openings in the middle cranial fossa are:
the optic canal
the superior orbital fissure
the foramen rotundum
the foramen ovale
the foramen spinosum
the venous (emissary sphenoidal) foramen (of Vesalius) (occasional)
the petrosal (innominate) foramen (occasional)
the foramen lacerum
the hiatus for the greater and lesser petrosal nerves
● The openings in the posterior cranial fossa are:
the foramen magnum   the jugular foramen
the internal acoustic meatus   the hypoglossal canal
the aqueduct of the   the condylar canal
    vestibule   the mastoid foramen
● For the contents of skull foramina see pages 25 and 223–225.

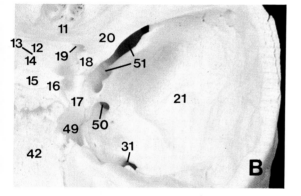

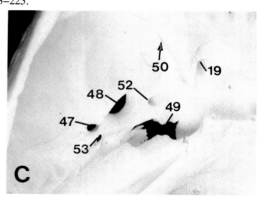

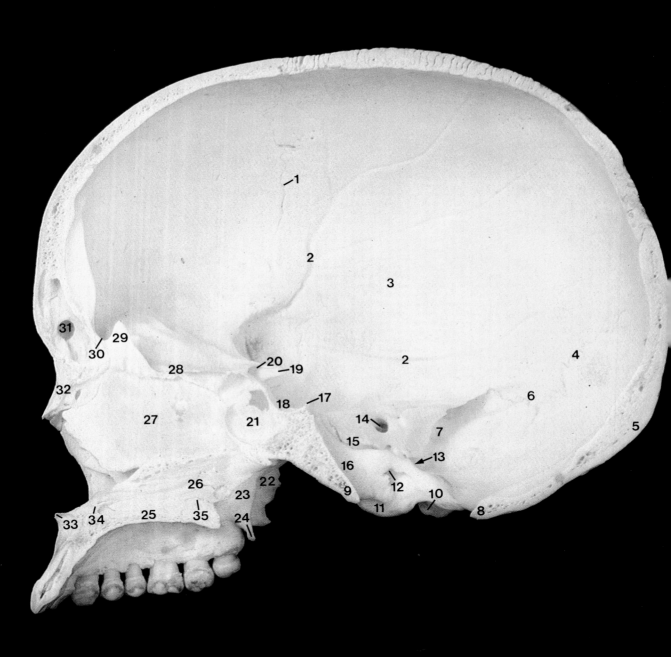

THE SKULL

Median sagittal section. The right half, with the bony nasal septum

1 Coronal suture
2 Grooves for middle meningeal vessels
3 Squamosal suture
4 Lambdoid suture
5 External occipital protuberance
6 Groove for transverse sinus
7 Groove for sigmoid sinus
8 Posterior ⎫
9 Anterior ⎬ margin of foramen magnum
10 Mastoid process
11 Occipital condyle
12 Hypoglossal canal
13 Jugular foramen
14 Internal acoustic meatus
15 Groove for inferior petrosal sinus
16 Clivus
17 Dorsum sellae
18 Pituitary fossa
19 Anterior clinoid process
20 Optic canal
21 Sphenoidal sinus
22 Lateral ⎫
23 Medial ⎬ pterygoid plate
24 Pterygoid hamulus
25 Hard palate
26 Vomer
27 Perpendicular plate ⎫
28 Cribriform plate ⎬ of ethmoid bone
29 Crista galli
30 Foramen caecum
31 Frontal sinus
32 Nasal bone
33 Anterior nasal spine
34 Nasal crest of maxilla
35 Nasal crest of palatine bone

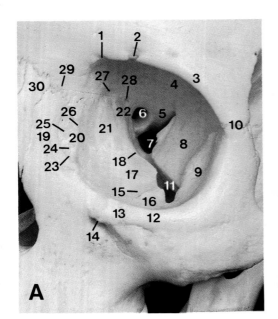

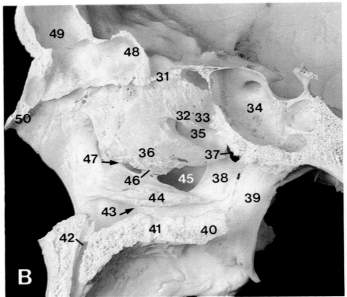

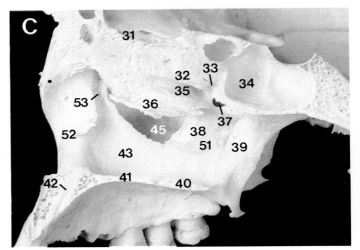

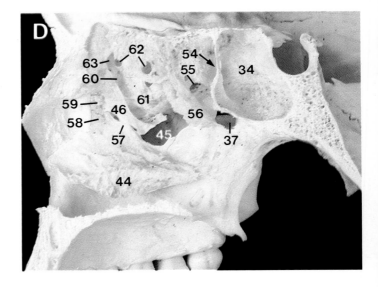

THE SKULL

The orbit and the nasal cavity

A **The left orbit, from the front, slightly left and above**

1 Frontal notch
2 Supra-orbital foramen
3 Supra-orbital margin
4 Orbital part of frontal bone ⎫
5 Lesser wing of sphenoid bone ⎬ forming roof
6 Optic canal
7 Superior orbital fissure
8 Greater wing of sphenoid ⎫
  bone ⎬ forming
9 Zygomatic bone ⎭ lateral wall
10 Frontozygomatic suture
11 Inferior orbital fissure
12 Infra-orbital margin
13 Zygomaticomaxillary suture
14 Infra-orbital foramen
15 Infra-orbital groove
16 Zygomatic bone ⎫
17 Maxilla ⎬ forming floor
18 Orbital process of palatine bone ⎭
19 Frontal process of maxilla ⎫
20 Lacrimal bone ⎬ forming
21 Orbital plate of ethmoid bone ⎬ medial wall
22 Body of sphenoid bone ⎭
23 Anterior lacrimal crest
24 Lacrimal groove
25 Fossa for lacrimal sac
26 Posterior lacrimal crest
27 Anterior ⎫
28 Posterior ⎬ ethmoidal foramen
29 Frontomaxillary suture
30 Nasal bone

● For further details of the bones of the orbit see pages 54–59.

B **The right half of the nasal cavity, lateral wall**
C **After removal of the inferior concha**
D **After removal of the middle concha**
E **Oblique view, from the front and the right, of the left side of a midline sagittal section of the skull** *(with the nasal septum removed)*

31 Cribriform plate of ethmoid bone
32 Superior nasal concha
33 Spheno-ethmoidal recess
34 Sphenoidal sinus
35 Superior meatus
36 Middle nasal concha
37 Sphenopalatine foramen
38 Perpendicular plate of palatine bone
39 Medial pterygoid plate
40 Horizontal plate of palatine bone
41 Palatine process of maxilla
42 Incisive canal
43 Inferior meatus
44 Inferior nasal concha
45 Maxillary hiatus
46 Uncinate process of ethmoid bone
47 Middle meatus
48 Crista galli
49 Frontal sinus
50 Nasal bone
51 Conchal crest of perpendicular plate of palatine bone
52 Conchal crest of maxilla
53 Nasolacrimal canal
54 Aperture of sphenoidal sinus into spheno-ethmoidal recess
55 Aperture of posterior ethmoidal air cell into superior meatus
56 Base of middle nasal concha
57 Ethmoidal process ⎫
58 Lacrimal process ⎬ of inferior nasal concha
59 Descending process of lacrimal bone
60 Semilunar hiatus

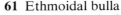

61 Ethmoidal bulla
62 Apertures of middle ethmoidal air cells
63 Frontonasal duct

● For further details of the bones of the nose see pages 54 and 60–63.

● In B the crista galli is large and the (left) frontal sinus has extended into it.

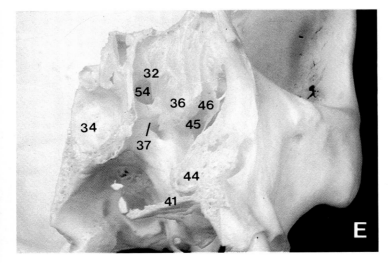

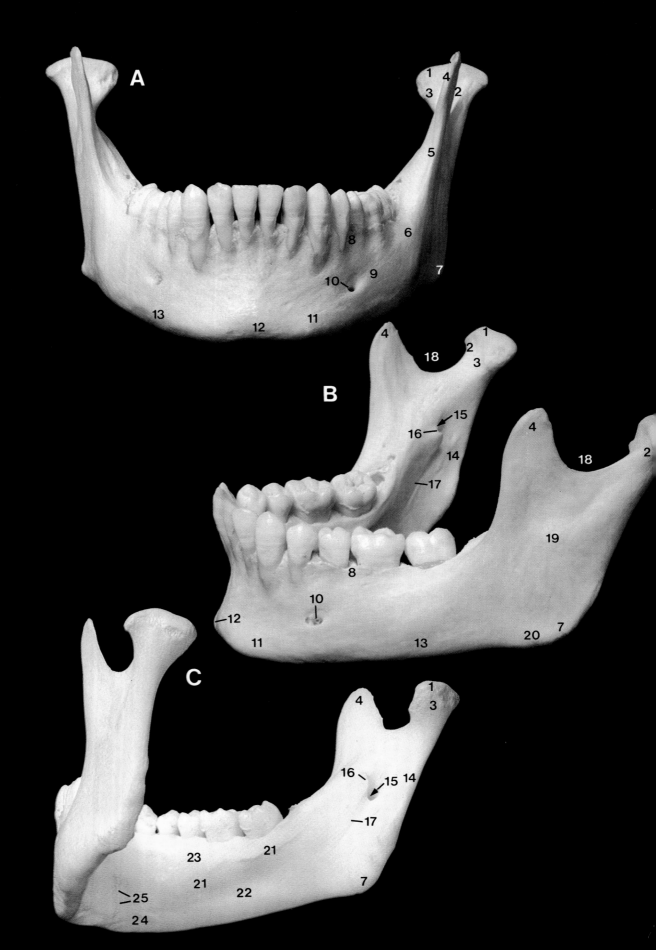

Bones of the Skull

THE MANDIBLE

A From the front
B From the left and above
C From the left and below
D From above

1 Head ⎫
2 Neck ⎬ forming condylar process
3 Pterygoid fovea ⎭
4 Coronoid process
5 Anterior border of ramus
6 Oblique line
7 Angle
8 Alveolar part
9 Body
10 Mental foramen
11 Mental tubercle
12 Mental protuberance
13 Base
14 Posterior border of ramus
15 Mandibular foramen
16 Lingula
17 Mylohyoid groove
18 Mandibular notch

19 Ramus
20 Inferior border of ramus
21 Mylohyoid line
22 Submandibular fossa
23 Sublingual fossa
24 Digastric fossa
25 Superior and inferior mental spines

● In this mandible the third molar teeth are unerupted.

● The main features of the mandible are:
the body with the lower teeth
the ramus passing upwards, with the mandibular foramen
   on its medial side
the coronoid process at the upper anterior end of the ramus
the condylar process (condyle) comprising the head and
   neck at the upper posterior end of the ramus
the angle at the lower posterior end of the ramus

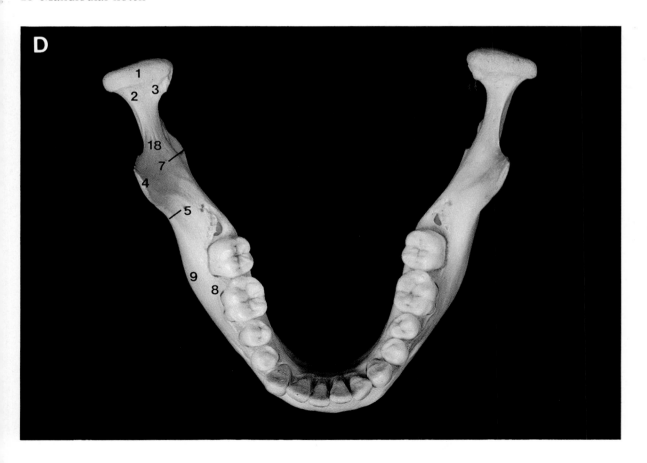

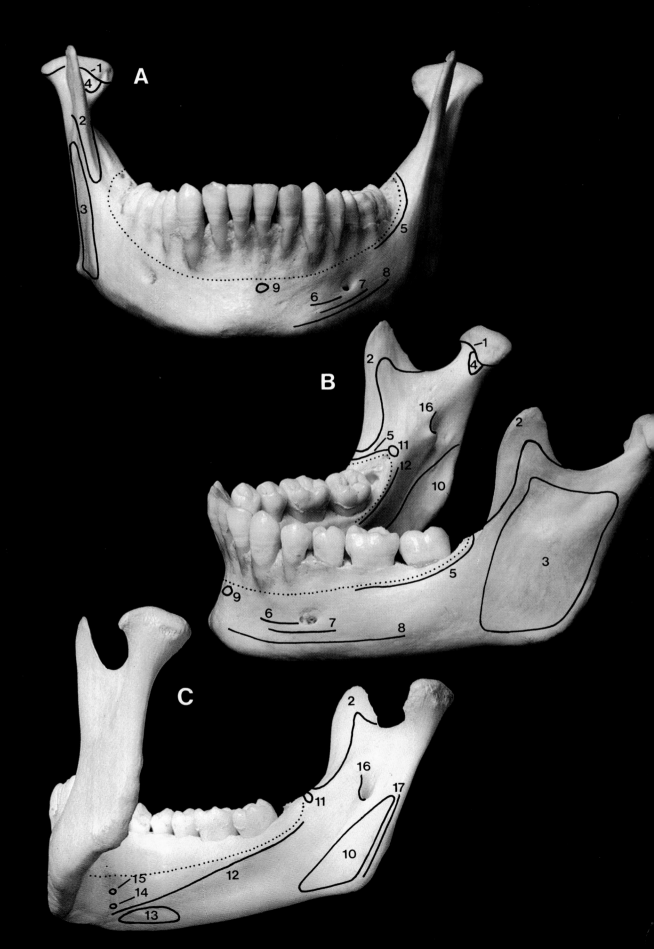

THE MANDIBLE

Muscle attachments

(The dotted line indicates the limit of attachment of the oral mucous membrane)

A From the front
B From the left and above
C From the left and below

  1 Capsule of temporomandibular joint
  2 Temporalis
  3 Masseter
  4 Lateral pterygoid
  5 Buccinator
  6 Depressor labii inferioris
  7 Depressor anguli oris
  8 Platysma
  9 Mentalis
10 Medial pterygoid
11 Pterygomandibular raphe and superior
     constrictor of pharynx
12 Mylohyoid
13 Anterior belly of digastric
14 Geniohyoid
15 Genioglossus
16 Sphenomandibular ligament
17 Stylomandibular ligament

**D The edentulous mandible of old age, from
   the right**

● Compare with the normal adult bone, as in B and C and
note that the angle between the ramus and body has become
more obtuse, and that alveolar bone has become resorbed so
that the mental foramen lies near the upper surface of the
edentulous body.

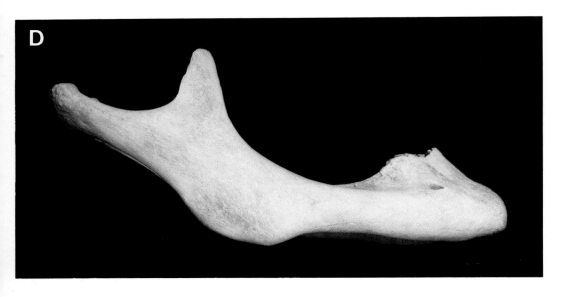

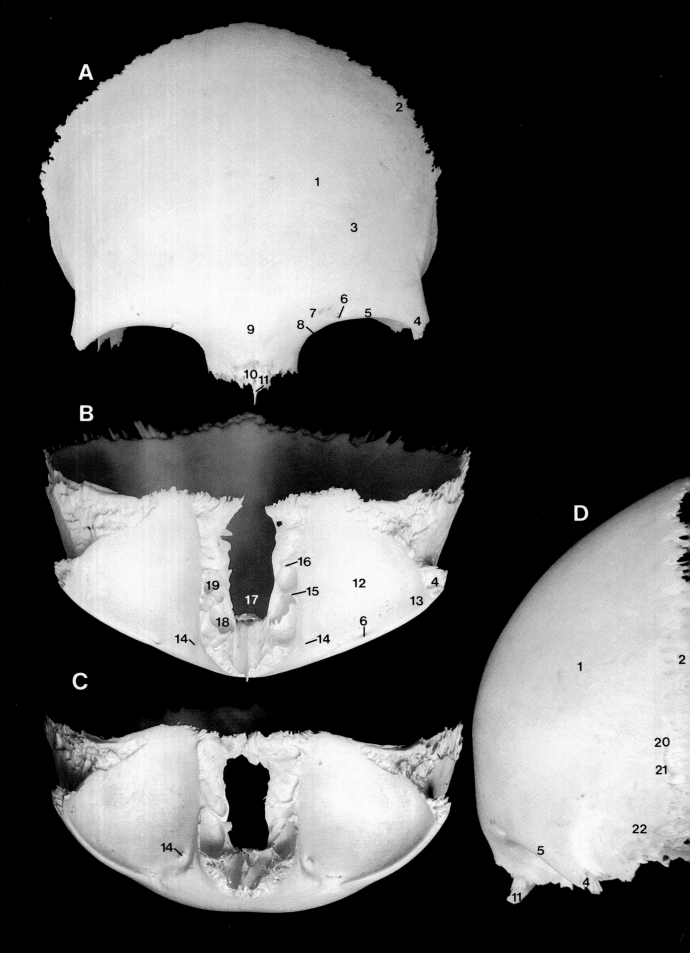

FRONTAL BONE

A   **External surface, from the front**
B & C **From below**
D   **External surface, from the left**
E   **Internal surface, from above and behind**
F   **External surface, from the front, showing the frontal suture**

1 Squamous part
2 Parietal margin
3 Frontal tuberosity
4 Zygomatic process
5 Supra-orbital margin
6 Supra-orbital foramen
7 Superciliary arch
8 Position of frontal notch or foramen
9 Glabella
10 Nasal part
11 Nasal spine
12 Orbital part
13 Fossa for lacrimal gland
14 Trochlear fovea (tubercle in C)

15 Anterior ethmoidal foramen
16 Posterior ethmoidal foramen
17 Ethmoidal notch
18 Frontal sinus
19 Roof of ethmoidal air cells
20 Superior temporal line
21 Inferior temporal line
22 Temporal surface
23 Frontal crest
24 Foramen caecum
25 Frontal (metopic) suture

● The main features of the frontal bone are:
    the squamous part curving upwards and backwards above the nose and orbits
    the orbital parts passing backwards as the roofs of the orbits
    the nasal part with the nasal spine passing downwards

● The frontal (metopic) suture is normally obliterated by the age of 8 years but occasionally persists into adult life, as in F.

● In C the orbital parts have become joined posteriorly.

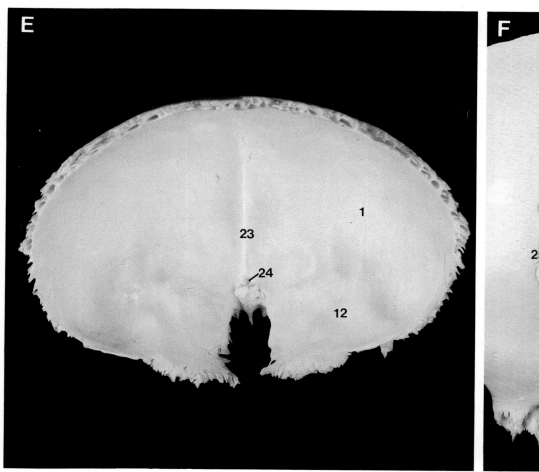

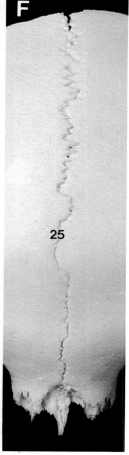

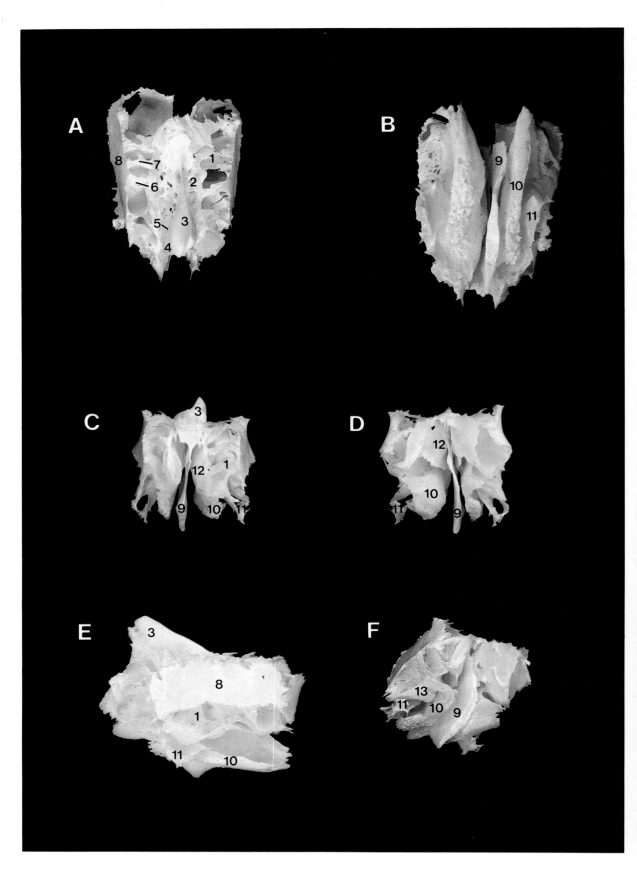

40

ETHMOID BONE

A **From above**
B **From below**
C **From the front**
D **From behind**
E **From the left**
F **From the left, below and behind**

1 Ethmoidal labyrinth and air cells
2 Cribriform plate
3 Crista galli
4 Ala of crista galli
5 Slit for anterior ethmoidal nerve and vessels
6 Groove for anterior ethmoidal nerve and vessels
7 Groove for posterior ethmoidal nerve and vessels
8 Orbital plate
9 Perpendicular plate
10 Middle nasal concha
11 Uncinate process
12 Superior nasal concha
13 Ethmoidal bulla

● The main features of the ethmoid bone are:
  the perpendicular plate with the crista galli at the upper end
  the cribriform plates
  the ethmoidal labyrinths (sinuses) containing air cells
  superior and middle nasal conchae on the medial side of each labyrinth

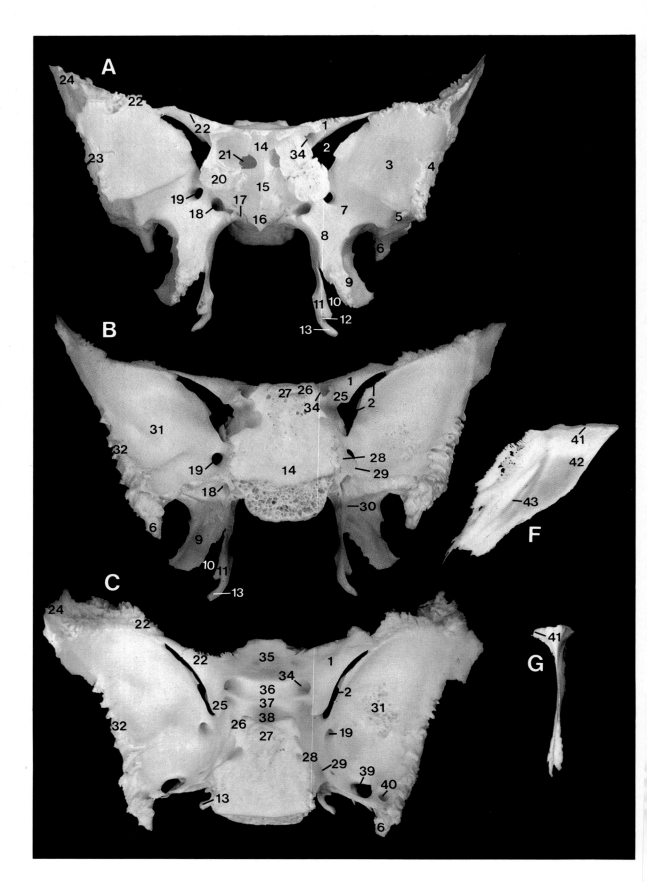

THE SPHENOID BONE

A From the front
B From behind
C From above and behind
D From below
E From the right

1 Lesser wing
2 Superior orbital fissure
3 Orbital surface ⎫
4 Temporal surface ⎪
5 Infratemporal crest ⎬ of greater wing
6 Spine ⎪
7 Maxillary surface ⎭
8 Pterygoid process
9 Lateral pterygoid plate
10 Pterygoid notch
11 Medial pterygoid plate
12 Groove of pterygoid hamulus
13 Pterygoid hamulus
14 Body
15 Crest
16 Rostrum
17 Vaginal process
18 Pterygoid canal
19 Foramen rotundum
20 Concha
21 Aperture of sphenoidal sinus
22 Frontal margin
23 Zygomatic margin
24 Parietal margin
25 Anterior clinoid process
26 Posterior clinoid process
27 Dorsum sellae
28 Carotid groove
29 Lingula
30 Scaphoid fossa

31 Cerebral surface of greater wing
32 Squamous margin
33 Groove for auditory tube
34 Optic canal
35 Jugum
36 Prechiasmatic groove
37 Tuberculum sellae
38 Pituitary fossa (sella turcica)
39 Foramen ovale
40 Foramen spinosum

● The main features of the sphenoid bone are:
the body containing the two sphenoidal sinuses with their
    apertures anteriorly
the lesser wings passing laterally with the optic canal between
    their roots
the greater wings passing laterally below the lesser wings
    with the superior orbital fissure between the lesser and
    greater wings and the foramen rotundum, ovale and
    spinosum within the greater wing
the pterygoid processes with medial and lateral pterygoid
    plates

● The posterior part of the body which joins the occipital
bone at the spheno-occipital synchondrosis (see page 67) is
commonly known as the basisphenoid.

THE VOMER

F From the left
G From behind

41 Ala
42 Posterior border
43 Groove for nasopalatine nerve and vessels

● The main features of the vomer are:
the alae that project laterally at the upper margin

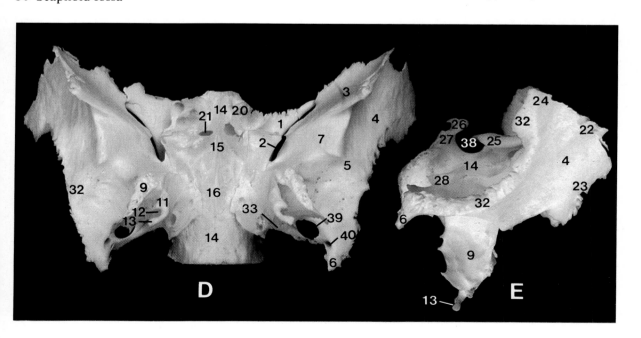

43

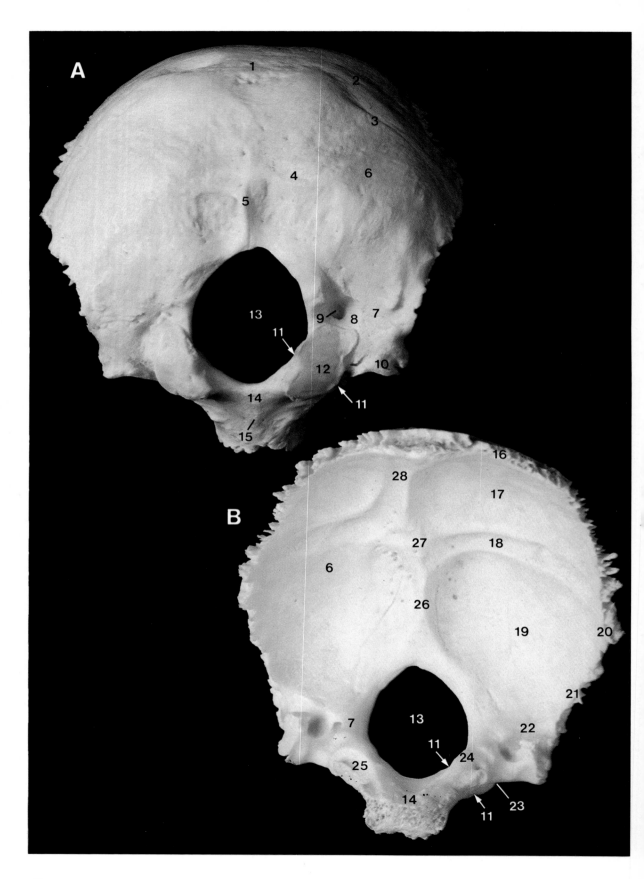

THE OCCIPITAL BONE

A External surface from below
B Internal surface
C External surface from the right and below

1 External occipital protuberance
2 Supreme nuchal line
3 Superior nuchal line
4 Inferior nuchal line
5 External occipital crest
6 Squamous part
7 Lateral part
8 Condylar fossa
9 Condylar canal
10 Jugular process
11 Hypoglossal canal
12 Condyle
13 Foramen magnum
14 Basilar part
15 Pharyngeal tubercle
16 Lambdoid margin
17 Cerebral fossa
18 Groove for transverse sinus
19 Cerebellar fossa
20 Lateral angle
21 Mastoid margin

22 Groove for sigmoid sinus
23 Jugular notch
24 Jugular tubercle
25 Groove for inferior petrosal sinus
26 Internal occipital crest
27 Internal occipital protuberance
28 Groove for superior sagittal sinus

● The main features of the occipital bone are:
 the foramen magnum
 the squamous part curving backwards and upwards behind the foramen
 the lateral parts, with condyles below, at the sides of the foramen
 the basilar part in front of the foramen

● The anterior end of the basilar part which joins the sphenoid bone at the spheno-occipital synchondrosis is commonly known as the basi-occiput.

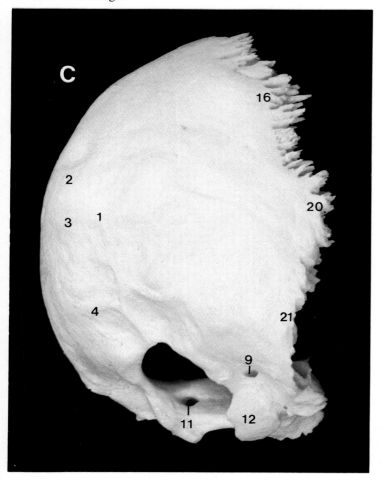

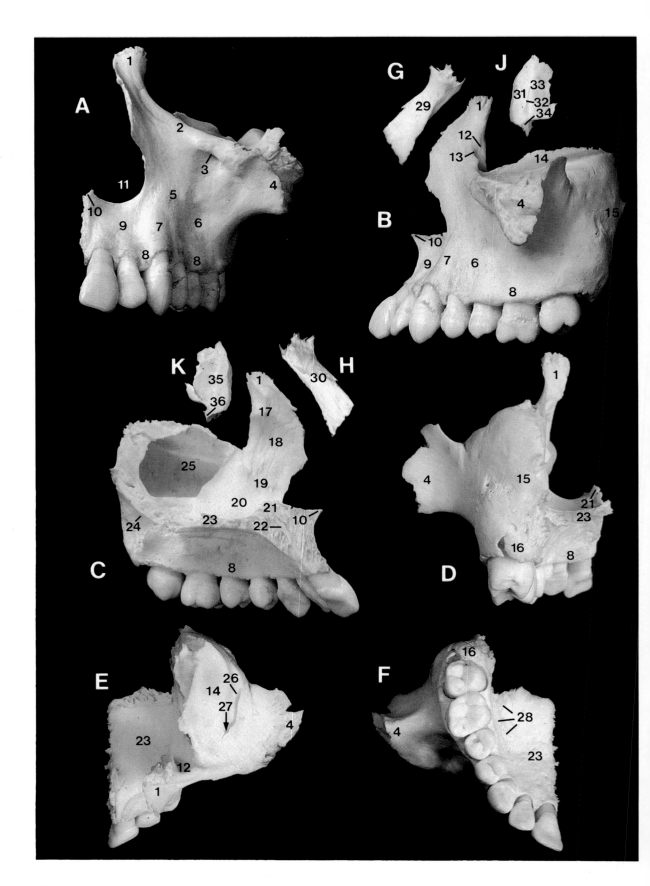

THE MAXILLA, left

A From the front
B From the lateral side
C From the medial side
D From behind
E From above
F From below

1 Frontal process
2 Infra-orbital margin
3 Infra-orbital foramen
4 Zygomatic process
5 Anterior surface
6 Canine fossa
7 Canine eminence
8 Alveolar process
9 Incisive fossa
10 Anterior nasal spine
11 Nasal notch
12 Lacrimal groove
13 Anterior lacrimal crest
14 Orbital surface
15 Infratemporal surface
16 Tuberosity
17 Ethmoidal crest
18 Middle meatus
19 Conchal crest
20 Inferior meatus
21 Nasal crest
22 Incisive canal
23 Palatine process
24 Greater palatine groove
25 Maxillary hiatus and sinus
26 Infra-orbital groove
27 Infra-orbital canal
28 Palatine grooves and spines

● The main features of the maxilla are:
the maxillary sinus with the hiatus in the medial wall
the alveolar process with the upper teeth
the frontal process passing upwards
the palatal process passing medially
the zygomatic process passing laterally

● In this specimen the third molar tooth is unerupted.

THE NASAL BONE, left

G From the lateral side
H From the medial side

29 Lateral surface and vascular foramen
30 Internal surface and ethmoidal groove

● The main features of the nasal bone are:
the smooth lateral surface
the ethmoidal groove on the internal surface

THE LACRIMAL BONE, left

J From the lateral side
K From the medial side

31 Lacrimal groove
32 Posterior lacrimal crest
33 Orbital surface
34 Lacrimal hamulus
35 Nasal surface
36 Descending process

● The main features of the lacrimal bone are:
the orbital (lateral) surface with the lacrimal groove at the
front
the descending process pointing downwards

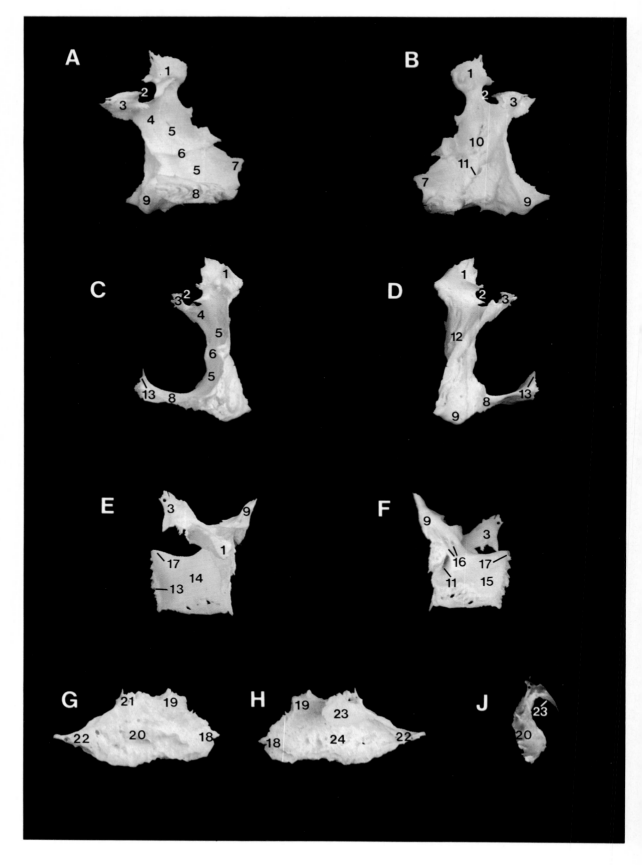

THE PALATINE BONE, left

A From the medial side
B From the lateral side
C From the front
D From behind
E From above
F From below

1 Orbital process
2 Sphenopalatine notch
3 Sphenoidal process
4 Ethmoidal crest
5 Perpendicular plate, nasal surface
6 Conchal crest
7 Maxillary process
8 Horizontal plate
9 Pyramidal process
10 Perpendicular plate, maxillary surface
11 Greater palatine groove
12 Perpendicular plate
13 Nasal crest
14 Horizontal plate, nasal surface
15 Horizontal plate, palatal surface
16 Lesser palatine canals
17 Posterior nasal spine

● The main features of the palatine bone are:
the perpendicular plate with the maxillary process passing
forwards at the lower end
the sphenoidal and orbital processes at the upper end of the
perpendicular plate with the sphenopalatine notch in
between
the horizontal plate passing medially at the lower end
the pyramidal process passing backwards at the lower end

THE INFERIOR NASAL CONCHA, left

G From the medial side
H From the lateral side
J From the front

18 Anterior end
19 Lacrimal process
20 Medial surface
21 Ethmoidal process
22 Posterior end
23 Maxillary process
24 Lateral surface

● The main features of the inferior nasal concha are:
the convex medial surface with a sharp posterior end
the lacrimal and ethmoidal processes passing upwards
the maxillary process passing downwards on the lateral side

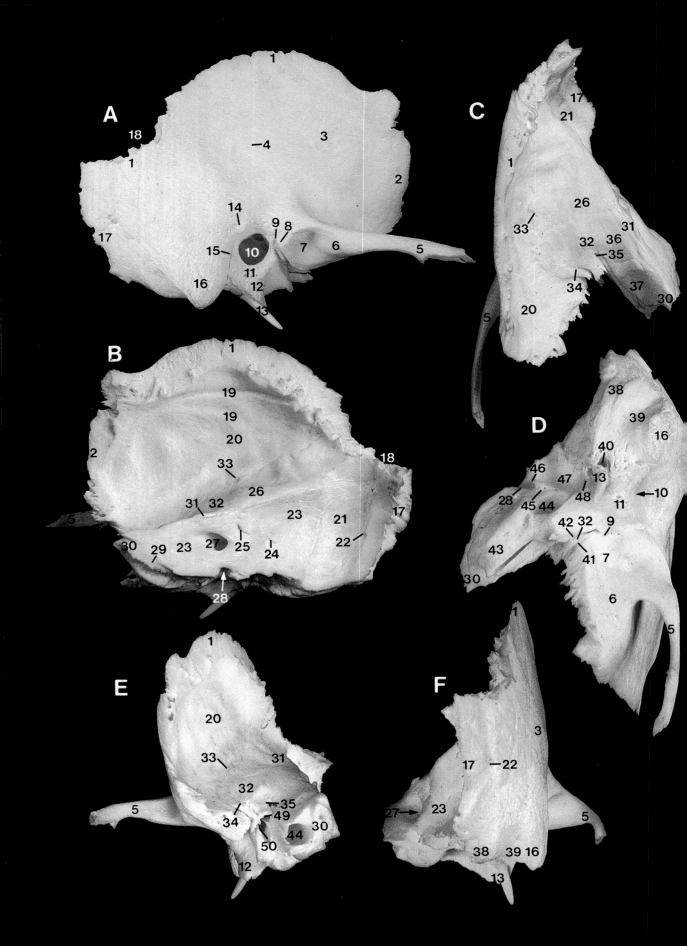

THE TEMPORAL BONE, right

A **From the lateral side**
B **From the medial side**
C **From above**
D **From below**
E **From the front**
F **From behind**
G **From the medial side and above**

 1 Parietal margin
 2 Sphenoidal margin
 3 Temporal surface of squamous part
 4 Groove for middle temporal artery
 5 Zygomatic process
 6 Articular tubercle
 7 Mandibular fossa
 8 Postglenoid tubercle
 9 Squamotympanic fissure
10 External acoustic meatus
11 Tympanic part
12 Sheath of styloid process
13 Styloid process
14 Suprameatal pit and spine (suprameatal triangle)
15 Tympanomastoid fissure
16 Mastoid process
17 Occipital margin
18 Parietal notch
19 Groove for parietal branches of middle meningeal vessels
20 Cerebral surface of squamous part
21 Groove for sigmoid sinus
22 Mastoid foramen
23 Posterior surface of petrous part
24 External opening of aqueduct of vestibule
25 Subarcuate fossa
26 Arcuate eminence
27 Internal acoustic meatus
28 External opening of cochlear canaliculus in jugular notch
29 Groove for inferior petrosal sinus
30 Apex of petrous part
31 Superior margin of petrous part and groove for superior petrosal sinus
32 Tegmen tympani
33 Petrosquamous fissure (upper part)
34 Hiatus and groove for lesser petrosal nerve
35 Hiatus and groove for greater petrosal nerve
36 Anterior surface of petrous part
37 Trigeminal impression
38 Occipital groove
39 Mastoid notch
40 Stylomastoid foramen
41 Petrosquamous fissure (lower part)
42 Petrotympanic fissure
43 Inferior surface of petrous part
44 Carotid canal
45 Tympanic canaliculus
46 Intrajugular process
47 Jugular fossa
48 Mastoid canaliculus
49 Semicanal for tensor tympani
50 Semicanal for auditory tube
51 Groove for petrosquamous sinus

● The main features of the temporal bone are:
the petrous part including the mastoid process
the squamous part passing upwards but including the mandibular fossa facing downwards and the zygomatic process passing forwards
the tympanic part surrounding the external acoustic meatus opening laterally
the internal acoustic meatus in the petrous part opening medially
the styloid process pointing downwards

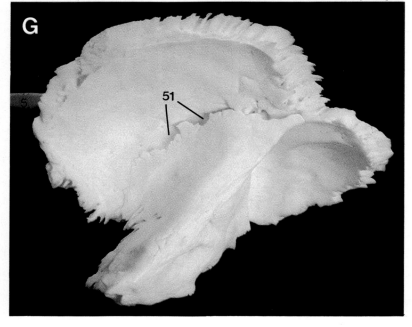

● The suprameatal triangle overlies the mastoid antrum which lies medially about 1.25 cm from the surface.

● The mastoid *foramen* transmits an emissary vein from the sigmoid sinus to the posterior auricular or occipital vein; the mastoid *canaliculus* (in the lateral part of the jugular fossa) transmits the auricular branch of the vagus nerve.

● The arcuate eminence overlies the anterior semicircular canal.

● For further details of the temporal bone and ear see pages 148–151.

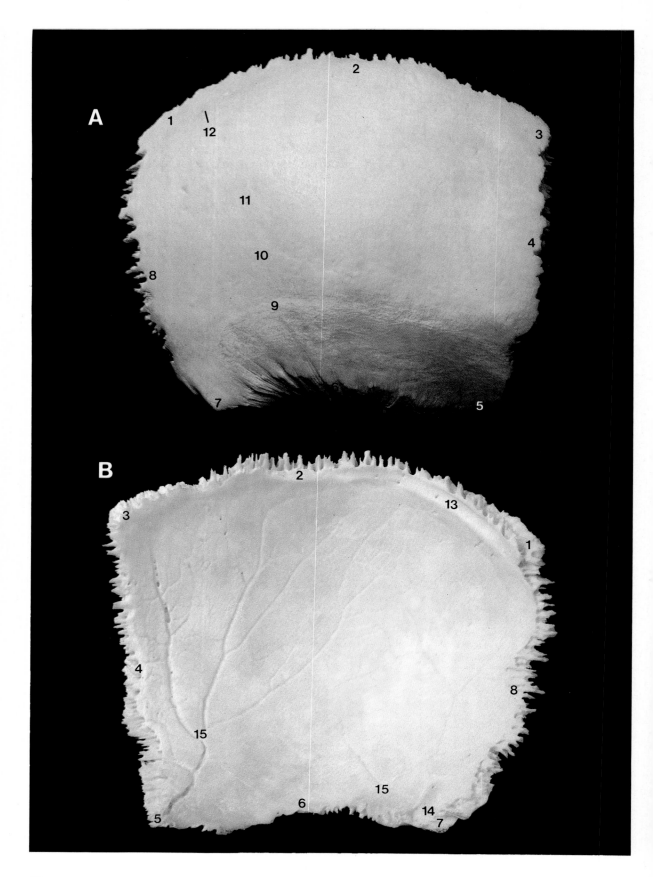

THE PARIETAL BONE, right

A External surface
B Internal surface

1 Occipital (posterosuperior) angle
2 Sagittal (superior) margin
3 Frontal (anterosuperior) angle
4 Frontal (anterior) margin
5 Sphenoidal (antero-inferior) angle
6 Squamous (inferior) margin
7 Mastoid (postero-inferior) angle
8 Occipital (posterior) margin
9 Inferior temporal line
10 Superior temporal line
11 Parietal tuberosity
12 Parietal foramen
13 Groove for part of superior sagittal sinus
14 Groove for sigmoid sinus at mastoid angle
15 Grooves for middle meningeal vessels

● The main features of the parietal bone are:
the convex external surface
the concave internal surface with grooves for the middle
meningeal vessels passing upwards and backwards, and
the groove for the sigmoid sinus at the mastoid
(postero-inferior) angle.

THE ZYGOMATIC BONE, left

C Lateral surface
D From the medial side
E From the front
F From behind

16 Frontal process
17 Temporal margin
18 Temporal process
19 Lateral surface
20 Maxillary margin
21 Zygomaticofacial foramen
22 Orbital margin
23 Orbital surface
24 Zygomatico-orbital foramen
25 Temporal surface
26 Zygomaticotemporal foramen
27 Sphenoidal margin
28 Marginal tubercle

● The main features of the zygomatic bone are:
the slightly convex lateral surface
the smoothly curved orbital margin and orbital surface
the frontal process passing upwards
the pointed temporal process passing backwards

● Official nomenclature does not recognise the margins of
the zygomatic bone, but these are helpful terms for
orientation.

● The marginal tubercle (Whitnall's tubercle) lies just inside
the orbital margin below the frontozygomatic suture, and it
can often be felt with the fingertip if not readily visible. It
receives the attachment of the lateral palpebral raphe (from
orbicularis oculi) and the lateral palpebral ligament.

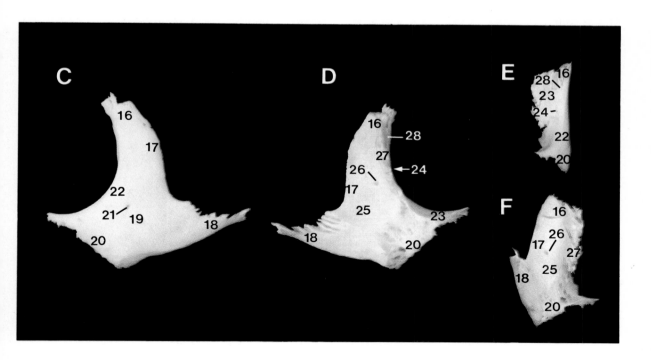

Skull Bone Articulations

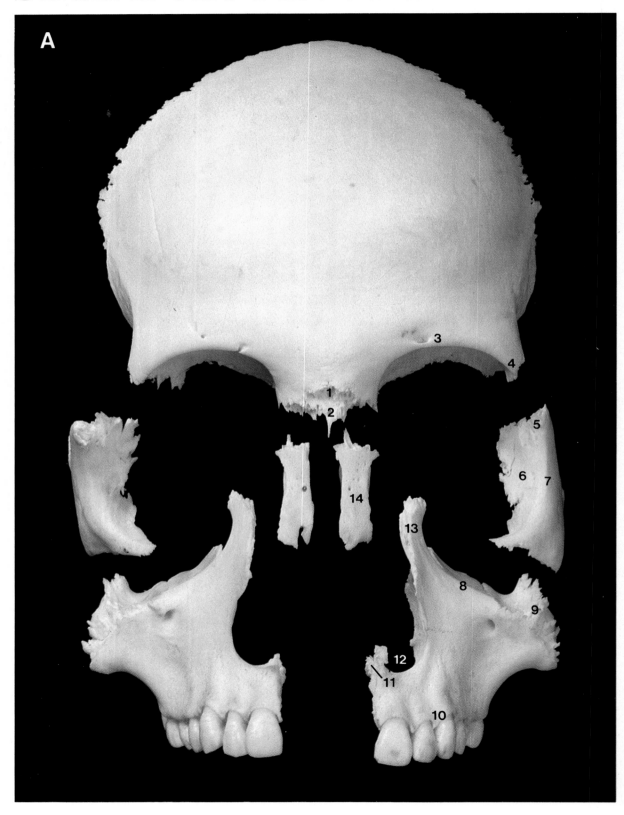

THE FACIAL SKELETON

The orbital and anterior nasal apertures

A & B The frontal, nasal and zygomatic bones and the maxillae, from the front, separated and articulated

 1 Nasal part
 2 Nasal spine
 3 Supra-orbital margin
 4 Zygomatic process
} of frontal bone

 5 Frontal process
 6 Orbital surface
 7 Orbital margin
} of zygomatic bone

 8 Infra-orbital margin
 9 Zygomatic process
10 Alveolar process
11 Anterior nasal spine
12 Nasal notch
13 Frontal process
14 Nasal bone
} of maxilla

● The orbital aperture (aditus of the orbit) is bounded above by the supra-orbital margin of the frontal bone, laterally by the zygomatic bone and the zygomatic process of the frontal bone, below by the zygomatic bone and the maxilla, and medially by the frontal bone and the anterior lacrimal crest of the frontal process of the maxilla.

● The anterior nasal (piriform) aperture is bounded largely by the two maxillae, with the lower margin of the nasal bones above.

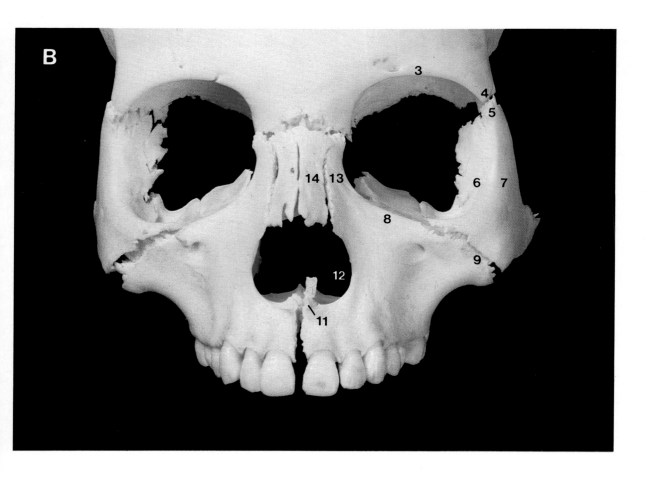

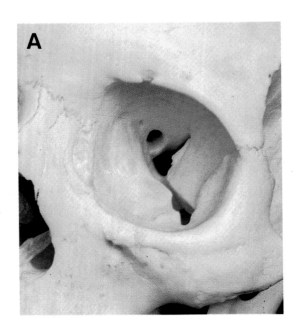

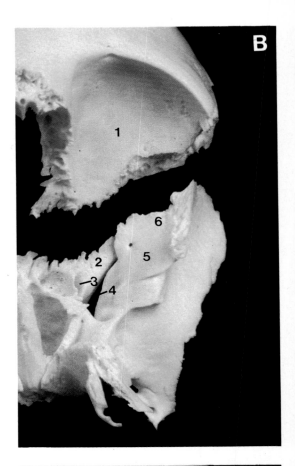

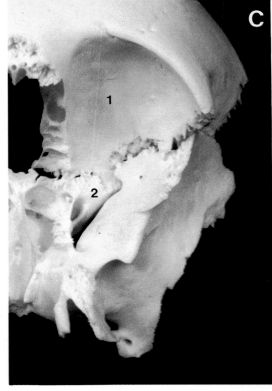

THE ORBIT

A The left orbit, from the front, left and above (as in 32A)

The roof of the left orbit

B & C Parts of the frontal and sphenoid bones, from below, separated and articulated

1 Orbital part of frontal bone
2 Lesser wing of sphenoid bone
3 Optic canal
4 Superior orbital fissure
5 Greater wing of sphenoid bone
6 Frontal margin of greater wing

● The roof of the orbit is formed mainly by the orbital part of the frontal bone, with the lesser wing of the sphenoid bone in the most posterior part. (The greater wing forms part of the lateral wall of the orbit – see below.)

The lateral wall of the left orbit

D & E Part of the sphenoid bone and the zygomatic bone, from the front (with the maxilla in E), separated and articulated

7 Lesser wing of sphenoid bone
8 Lateral wall of body
9 Pterygoid process
10 Foramen rotundum
11 Superior orbital fissure
12 Orbital surface of greater wing
13 Zygomatic margin
14 Orbital surface ⎫
15 Frontal process ⎪
16 Marginal tubercle ⎬ of zygomatic bone
17 Orbital margin ⎭
18 Infra-orbital margin ⎫ of maxilla
19 Orbital surface ⎬
20 Inferior orbital fissure

● The lateral wall of the orbit is formed by the orbital surfaces of the greater wing of the sphenoid and the zygomatic bones. (The zygomatic bone also forms part of the floor of the orbit, with the maxilla – see next page.)

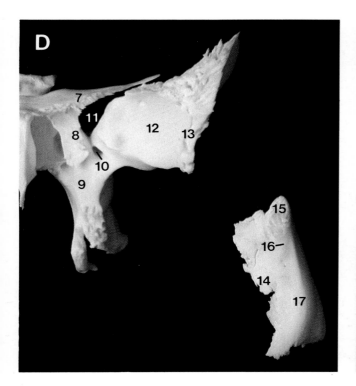

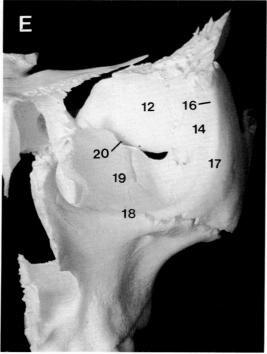

THE ORBIT

The floor of the left orbit

A & B **The left maxilla and zygomatic bone, from above and in front, separated and articulated** *(Note that the orbital process of the palatine bone remains adherent to this maxilla)*

C **The left maxilla and palatine bone, from above and in front, articulated**

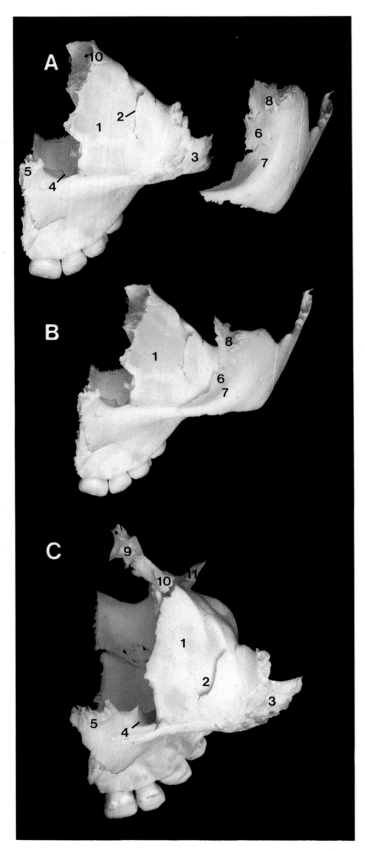

1 Orbital surface
2 Infra-orbital groove
3 Zygomatic process } of maxilla
4 Lacrimal groove
5 Frontal process

6 Orbital surface
7 Orbital margin } of zygomatic bone
8 Frontal process

9 Sphenoidal process
10 Orbital process } of palatine bone
11 Pyramidal process

● The floor of the orbit is formed by the orbital surfaces of the maxilla and zygomatic bone, with the orbital process of the palatine bone in the most posterior part.

The medial wall of the left orbit

D & E The lacrimal and ethmoid bones and the maxilla, from the left, separated and articulated *(The sphenoid bone, part of whose body forms the most posterior part of the medial wall, is not included. See page 57)*

12 Frontal process ⎫
13 Anterior lacrimal crest ⎬ of maxilla
14 Lacrimal groove ⎪
15 Orbital surface ⎭
16 Lacrimal groove ⎫
17 Posterior lacrimal crest ⎬ of lacrimal bone
18 Orbital surface ⎪
19 Lacrimal hamulus ⎭
20 Orbital plate of ethmoid bone
21 Nasolacrimal canal
22 Fossa for lacrimal sac

● The medial wall of the orbit begins at the anterior lacrimal crest of the frontal process of the maxilla. The lacrimal grooves of this process and of the lacrimal bone form the fossa for the lacrimal sac, and behind the posterior lacrimal crest lies the rest of the orbital surface of the lacrimal bone. The orbital plate of the ethmoid bone then forms much of the medial wall, with a small part of the body of the sphenoid (not shown here but seen in A on page 57) as the most posterior part of this wall.

● The upper parts of the lacrimal grooves of the maxilla and lacrimal bone form the fossa for the lacrimal sac.

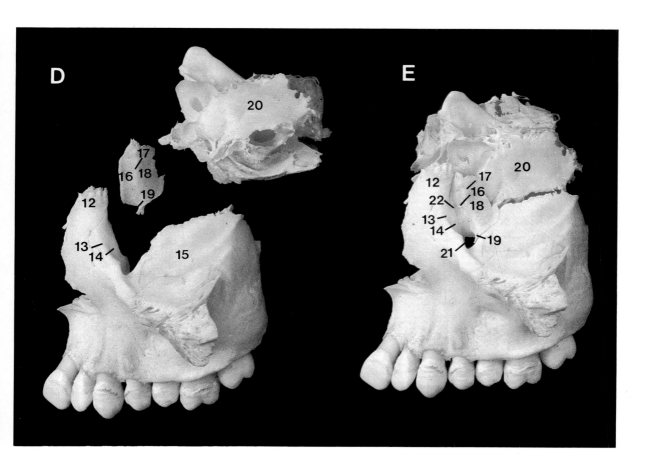

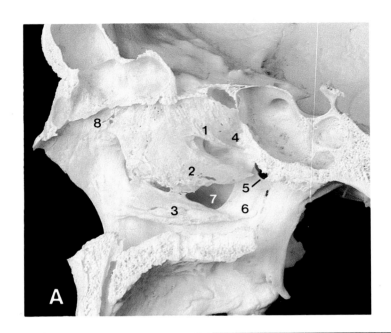

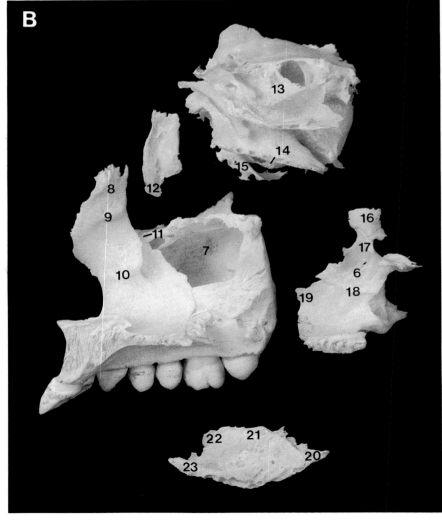

THE NOSE

The roof, floor and lateral wall of the right half of the nasal cavity

A   In the intact skull (as in B on page 32)
B   The right maxilla, lacrimal and palatine bones, inferior concha and the ethmoid bone, from the left
C   Maxilla with lacrimal and palatine bones and inferior concha
D & E The ethmoid bone and inferior concha, separated and articulated

1 Superior ⎫
2 Middle ⎬ nasal concha
3 Inferior ⎭
4 Spheno-ethmoidal recess
5 Sphenopalatine foramen
6 Perpendicular plate of palatine bone
7 Maxillary hiatus
8 Frontal process ⎫
9 Ethmoidal crest ⎬ of maxilla
10 Conchal crest ⎬
11 Lacrimal groove ⎭
12 Descending process of lacrimal bone
13 Left ethmoidal labyrinth ⎫
14 Right ethmoidal bulla ⎬ of ethmoid bone
15 Right uncinate process ⎭
16 Orbital process ⎫
17 Ethmoidal crest ⎬ of palatine bone
18 Conchal crest ⎬
19 Maxillary process ⎭
20 Posterior end ⎫
21 Ethmoidal process ⎬ of inferior concha
22 Lacrimal process ⎬
23 Anterior end ⎭

● In A the (left) frontal sinus is large and has extended into the crista galli.

● The roof of each half of the nasal cavity is formed centrally by the cribriform plate of the ethmoid bone, with anteriorly the nasal bone and the nasal spine of the frontal bone, and posteriorly the body of the sphenoid bone overlapped by the ala of the vomer and the sphenoidal process of the palatine bone.

● The floor is formed by the palatine process of the maxilla and the horizontal plate of the palatine bone.

● The medial wall is the nasal septum, whose bony part consists of the perpendicular plate of the ethmoid bone and (behind) the vomer (with the nasal crests of the maxilla and the palatine bone at the very base), and (in front) the septal cartilage.

● The lateral wall consists of the medial surface of the maxilla with the large maxillary hiatus being reduced in size by the overlapping of the lacrimal and ethmoid bones (above), the palatine bone (behind) and the inferior concha (below) (see next page).

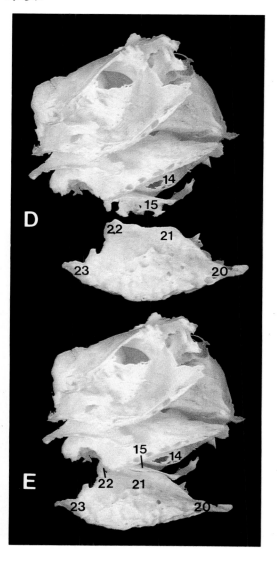

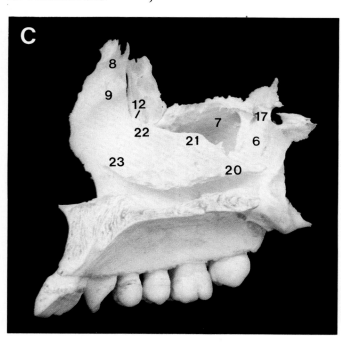

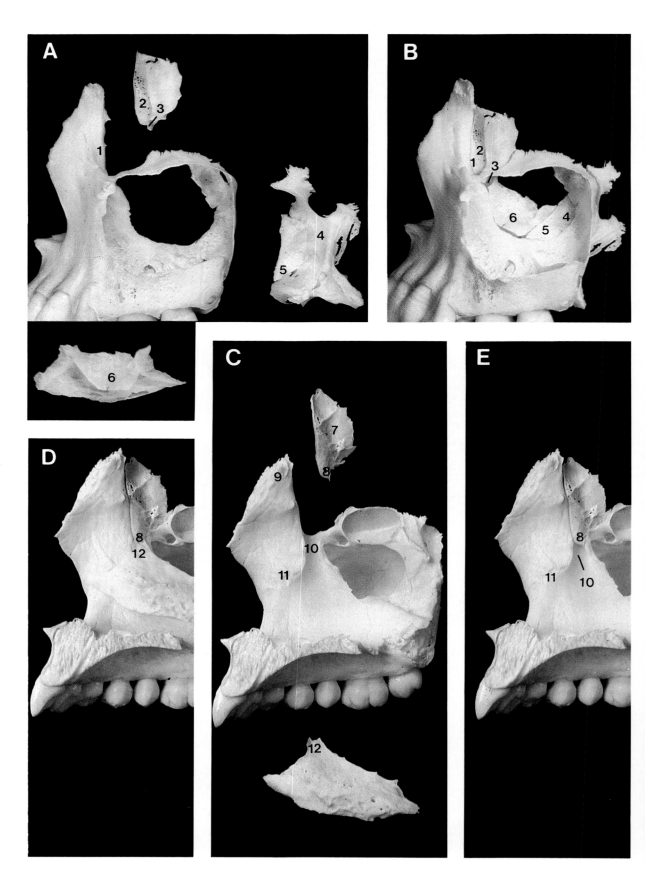

THE NOSE

The maxillary hiatus

A & B The left maxillary hiatus, from the left
(after removal of much of the lateral wall and orbital surface of the maxilla, with the lacrimal and palatine bones and inferior concha, separated and articulated)

1 Lacrimal groove of maxilla
2 Lacrimal groove ⎫
3 Descending process ⎬ of lacrimal bone
4 Perpendicular plate ⎫
5 Maxillary process ⎬ of palatine bone
6 Maxillary process of inferior concha

● The lacrimal and palatine bones and the inferior concha articulate with the maxilla to reduce the size of the hiatus. (The ethmoid bone which closes the upper part of the hiatus is not shown.)

The nasolacrimal canal

C The right maxilla, lacrimal bone and inferior concha, from the medial side, separated
D The maxilla, lacrimal bone and inferior concha, articulated
E The maxilla and lacrimal bone, articulated

7 Nasal surface ⎫
8 Descending process ⎬ of lacrimal bone
9 Frontal process ⎫
10 Lacrimal groove ⎬ of maxilla
11 Conchal crest ⎭
12 Lacrimal process of inferior concha

● The lacrimal groove of the maxilla is converted into the nasolacrimal canal by articulation with the descending process of the lacrimal bone, and the lower part of the canal is completed by the lacrimal process of the inferior concha.

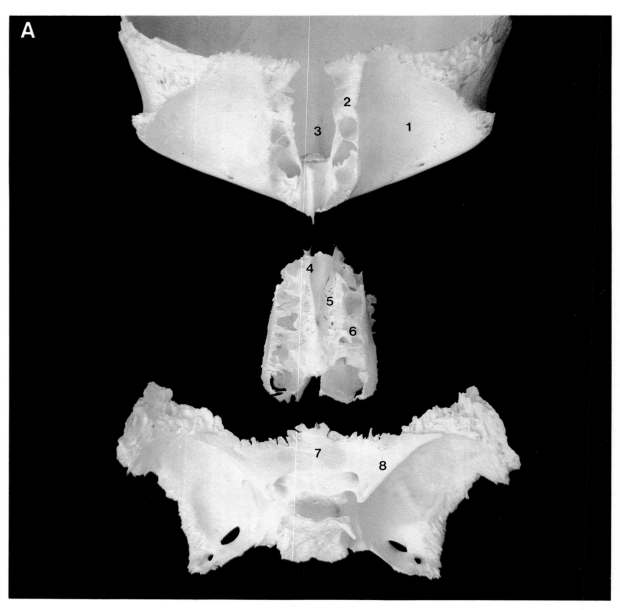

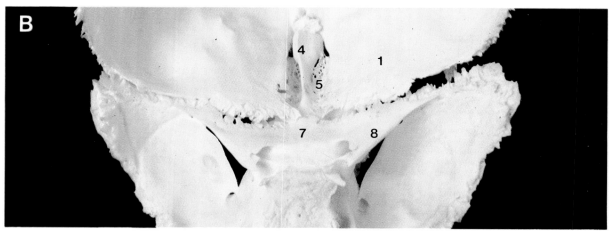

THE BASE OF THE SKULL

The anterior cranial fossa

A The frontal, ethmoid and sphenoid bones, from above and behind, with the frontal bone rotated forwards

B From above and behind, articulated

1 Orbital part of frontal bone
2 Roof of ethmoidal air cells
3 Ethmoidal notch
4 Crista galli
5 Cribriform plate of ethmoid bone
6 Ethmoidal labyrinth and air cells
7 Jugum of sphenoid bone
8 Lesser wing of sphenoid bone

● The medial part of the orbital part of the frontal bone forms the roof of the ethmoidal air cells, while the anterior wall of the body of the sphenoid completes the posterior wall of the ethmoidal labyrinth.

● The anterior cranial fossa is formed by the orbital parts of the frontal bone, the cribriform plates of the ethmoid bone with the crista galli, and the lesser wings and jugum of the sphenoid bone.

● The middle cranial fossa (see page 66) consists of a central part, formed by the body of the sphenoid bone, and right and left lateral parts each formed by the greater wing of the sphenoid and the squamous and petrous parts of the temporal bone.

● The posterior cranial fossa (see page 66) is formed by the basilar, lateral and lower squamous parts of the occipital bone, the petrous and mastoid parts of the temporal bones, a small part of the mastoid angles of the parietal bones (not shown here but see page 29), and the dorsum sellae and posterior part of the body of the sphenoid bone.

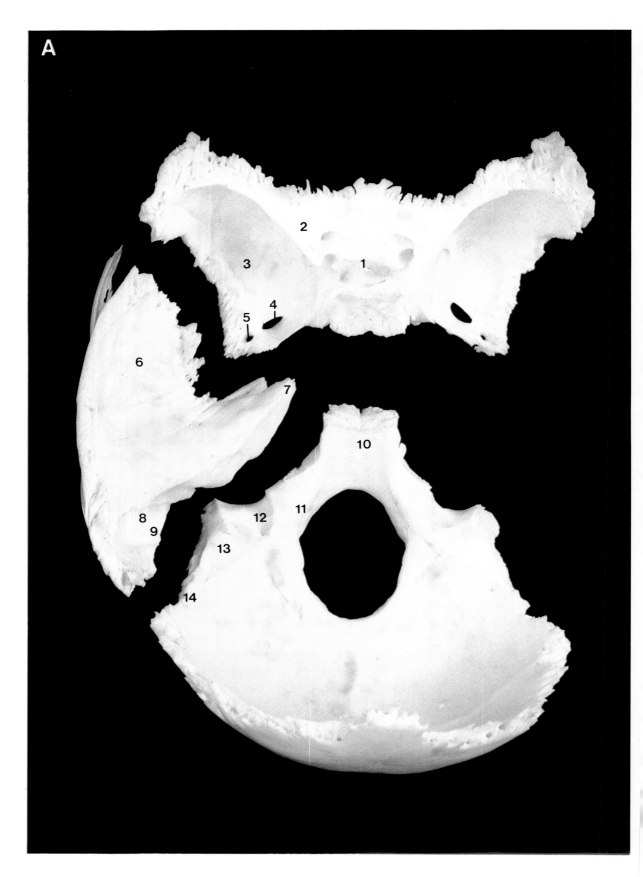

THE BASE OF THE SKULL

The middle and posterior cranial fossae

**A & B The sphenoid, left temporal and occipital
bones, from above, separated and
articulated** *(The right temporal bone has
been omitted)*

1 Body ⎫
2 Lesser wing ⎪
3 Greater wing ⎬ of sphenoid bone
4 Foramen ovale ⎪
5 Foramen spinosum ⎭
6 Squamous part of temporal bone
7 Apex ⎫ of petrous part
8 Groove for sigmoid sinus ⎬ of temporal
9 Occipital margin ⎭ bone
10 Basilar part ⎫
11 Lateral part ⎪
12 Jugular notch ⎬ of occipital bone
13 Groove for sigmoid sinus ⎪
14 Mastoid margin ⎭
15 Foramen lacerum

16 Sphenopetrosal synchondrosis
17 Spheno-occipital synchondrosis
18 Petro-occipital suture and groove for inferior
petrosal sinus
19 Jugular foramen
20 Occipitomastoid suture
21 Sphenosquamosal suture

● For notes on the bones of the middle and posterior cranial
fossae see page 65.

● The junction between the basilar part of the occipital bone
(basi-occiput) and the central posterior part of the sphenoid
bone (basisphenoid) is a synchondrosis which becomes a
complete bony union by the age of 25 years.

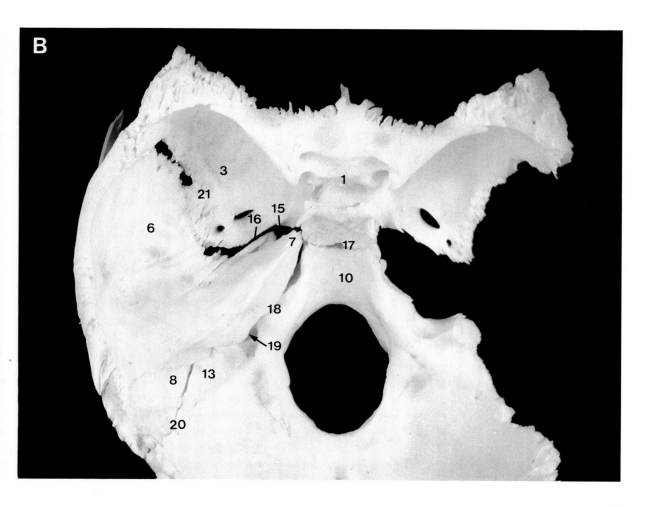

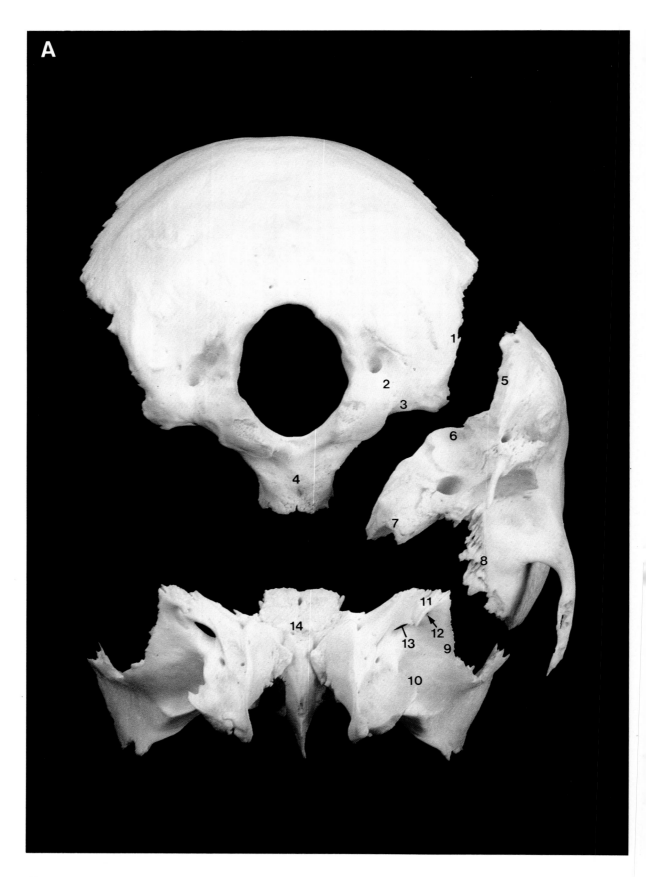

THE BASE OF THE SKULL

The external surface of the posterior part of the base

A & B The sphenoid, right temporal and occipital bones, from below, separated and articulated (*The left temporal bone has been omitted*)

 1 Mastoid margin
 2 Lateral part ⎫ of occipital bone
 3 Jugular notch
 4 Basilar part ⎭
 5 Occipital margin ⎫ of petrous part of
 6 Jugular notch ⎬ temporal bone
 7 Apex ⎭
 8 Sphenoidal margin of squamous part of temporal bone
 9 Squamous margin ⎫
10 Greater wing
11 Spine
12 Foramen spinosum ⎬ of sphenoid bone
13 Foramen ovale
14 Body ⎭
15 Occipitomastoid suture
16 Jugular foramen
17 Petro-occipital suture
18 Foramen lacerum
19 Spheno-occipital synchondrosis
20 Sphenopetrosal synchondrosis and groove for auditory tube
21 Sphenosquamosal suture

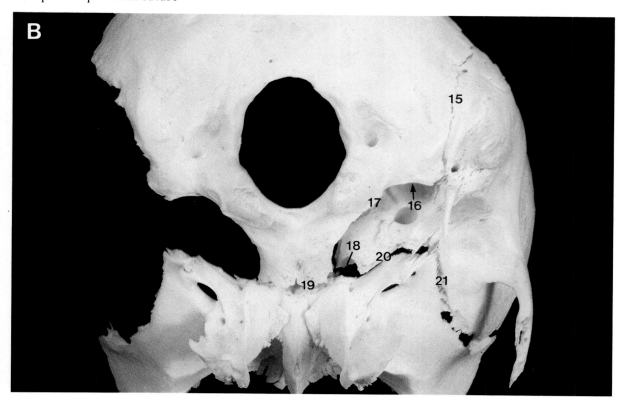

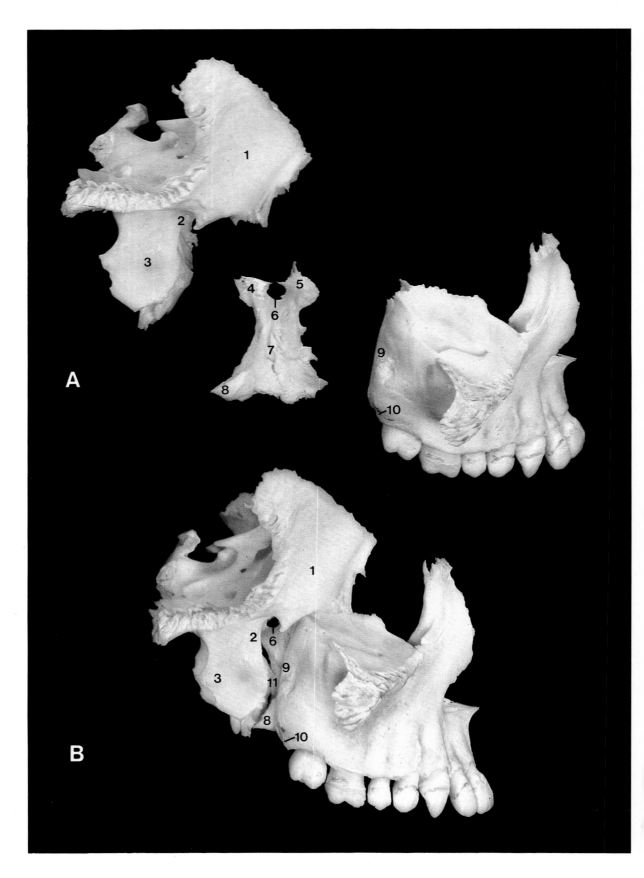

THE PTERYGOPALATINE FOSSA

The formation of the right pterygopalatine fossa

A & B The right maxilla and the palatine and sphenoid bones, from the right, separated and articulated

1 Temporal surface of greater wing
2 Pterygoid process
3 Lateral pterygoid plate
} of sphenoid bone

4 Sphenoidal process
5 Orbital process
6 Sphenopalatine notch
7 Perpendicular plate
8 Pyramidal process
} of palatine bone

9 Infratemporal surface
10 Tuberosity
} of maxilla

11 Pterygomaxillary fissure

● The medial wall of the pterygopalatine fossa is formed by the perpendicular plate of the palatine bone. The sphenopalatine notch at the upper end of the plate is converted into a foramen by the overlying body of the sphenoid bone (not shown in this illustration).

● The anterior wall of the fossa is formed by the infratemporal (posterior) surface of the maxilla.

● The posterior wall of the fossa is formed by the pterygoid process of the sphenoid bone.

● Laterally the pterygomaxillary fissure forms the communication between the pterygopalatine fossa and the infratemporal fossa.

● The pyramidal process of the palatine bone articulates with the tuberosity of the maxilla and fills in the triangular gap between the lower ends of the medial and lateral pterygoid plates (see pages 23 & 73).

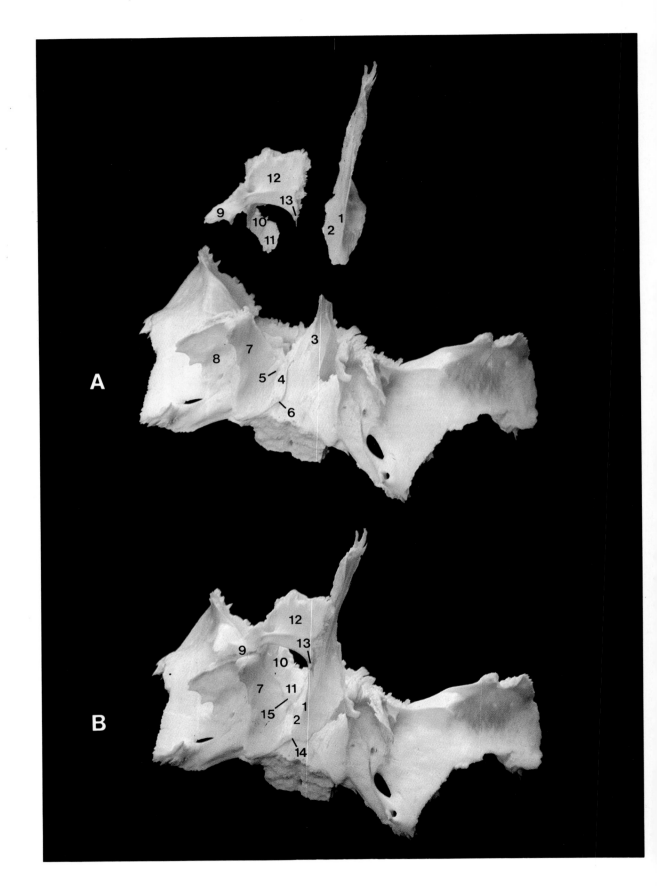

THE POSTERIOR NASAL APERTURE

A & B **The sphenoid bone with the right palatine bone and the vomer from below, right and behind, separated and articulated**

1 Posterior border ⎫
2 Ala ⎬ of vomer
3 Rostrum
4 Vaginal process
5 Groove that becomes palatovaginal canal when articulated with sphenoidal process of palatine bone
6 Groove that becomes vomerovaginal canal when articulated with ala of vomer
7 Medial pterygoid plate
8 Lateral pterygoid plate
9 Pyramidal process ⎫
10 Perpendicular plate ⎪
11 Sphenoidal process ⎬ of palatine bone
12 Horizontal plate ⎪
13 Posterior nasal spine ⎭
14 Vomerovaginal canal
15 Palatovaginal canal

● The posterior border of the vomer separates the two posterior nasal apertures (choanae), which are bounded below by the posterior border of the horizontal plate of the palatine bone, laterally by the medial pterygoid plate, and above by the body and vaginal process of the sphenoid bone and the ala of the vomer.

● A groove on the *lower* surface of the vaginal process of the sphenoid bone is converted into the palatovaginal canal by articulation with the upper surface of the sphenoidal process of the palatine bone.

● The vomerovaginal canal lies between the *upper* surface of the vaginal process of the sphenoid bone and the ala of the vomer. Anteriorly the vomerovaginal canal joins the palatovaginal canal.

● The pyramidal process of the palatine bone fills in the gap between the lower ends of the medial and lateral pterygoid plates (see page 22, B).

The Fetal Skull

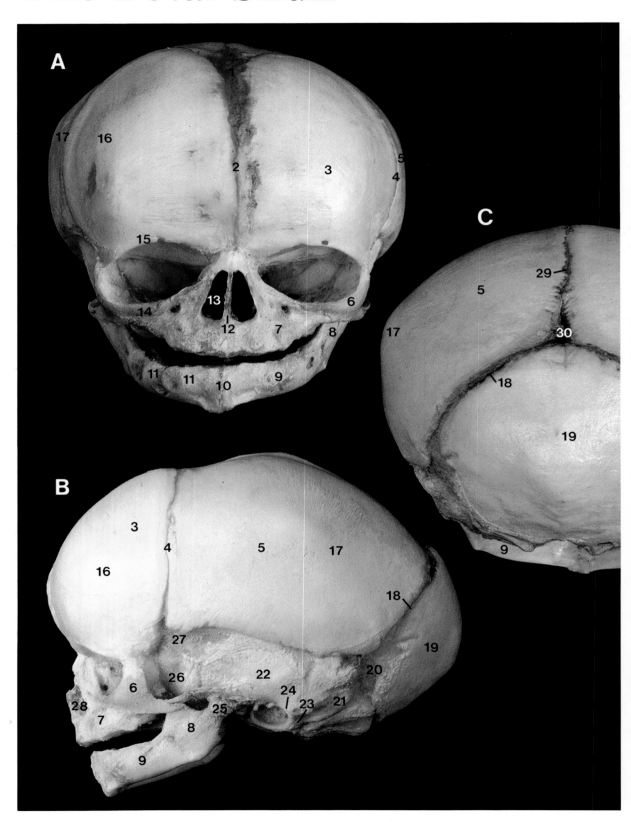

THE FETAL SKULL

The skull of a full-term fetus

A **From the front**
B **From the left**
C **From behind (left side)**
D **From above**

1 Anterior fontanelle
2 Frontal (metopic) suture
3 Half (squamous part) of frontal bone
4 Coronal suture
5 Parietal bone
6 Zygomatic bone
7 Maxilla
8 Ramus ⎫
9 Body ⎬ of mandible
10 Symphysis menti
11 Elevations over deciduous teeth
12 Nasal septum
13 Anterior nasal aperture
14 Infra-orbital margin
15 Supra-orbital margin
16 Frontal tuberosity
17 Parietal tuberosity

18 Lambdoid suture
19 Occipital bone
20 Mastoid (posterolateral) fontanelle
21 Petrous part ⎫
22 Squamous part ⎬ of temporal bone
23 Stylomastoid foramen
24 Tympanic ring
25 Condylar process of mandible
26 Greater wing of sphenoid bone
27 Sphenoidal (anterolateral) fontanelle
28 Septal cartilage
29 Sagittal suture
30 Posterior fontanelle

● The small sizes of the nasal cavity and the maxillary sinuses and the lack of erupted teeth all contribute to the face at birth forming a relatively smaller proportion of the cranium than in the adult (about one-eighth compared with one-half).

● The sphenoidal and posterior fontanelles close within three months of birth, the mastoid fontanelle at one year and the anterior fontanelle at about 18 months.

● The mastoid process does not develop until the second year, so that before then the stylomastoid foramen and the facial nerve are relatively near the surface and unprotected.

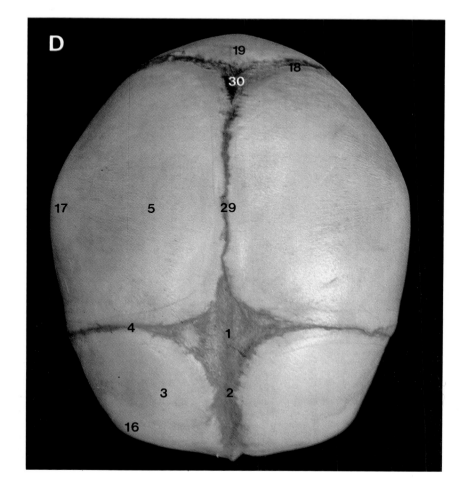

Vertebrae

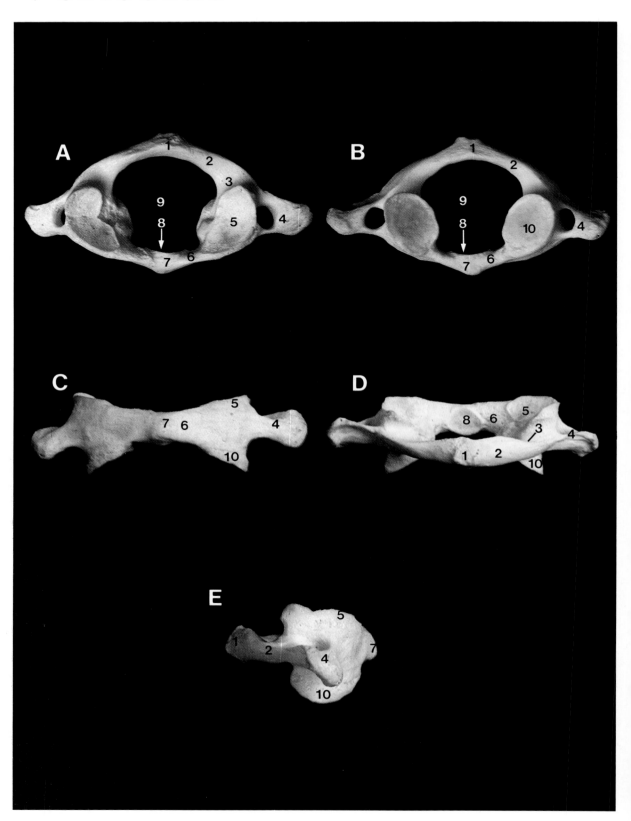

THE ATLAS (First Cervical Vertebra)

A From above
B From below
C From the front
D From behind
E From the right

1 Posterior tubercle
2 Posterior arch
3 Groove for vertebral artery
4 Transverse process and foramen
5 Lateral mass with superior articular facet
6 Anterior arch
7 Anterior tubercle
8 Facet for dens of axis
9 Vertebral foramen
10 Lateral mass with inferior articular facet

● All seven cervical vertebrae have a foramen in their transverse processes. This feature distinguishes them from the vertebrae of all other parts of the vertebral column.
● The typical cervical vertebrae are the third to the sixth (page 80).
● The first cervical vertebra (the atlas – this page), the second (the axis – page 78) and the seventh (vertebra prominens – page 80) have characteristic features.
● The atlas is the only vertebra that has no body – it is represented by the dens of axis.
● The superior articular facets are concave and kidney shaped.
● The inferior articular facets are round and almost flat.
● The anterior arch is straighter and shorter than the posterior arch, and bears on its posterior surface the articular facet for the dens of the axis (median atlanto-axial joint).
● The atlas has no spinous process; instead there is a small posterior tubercle.

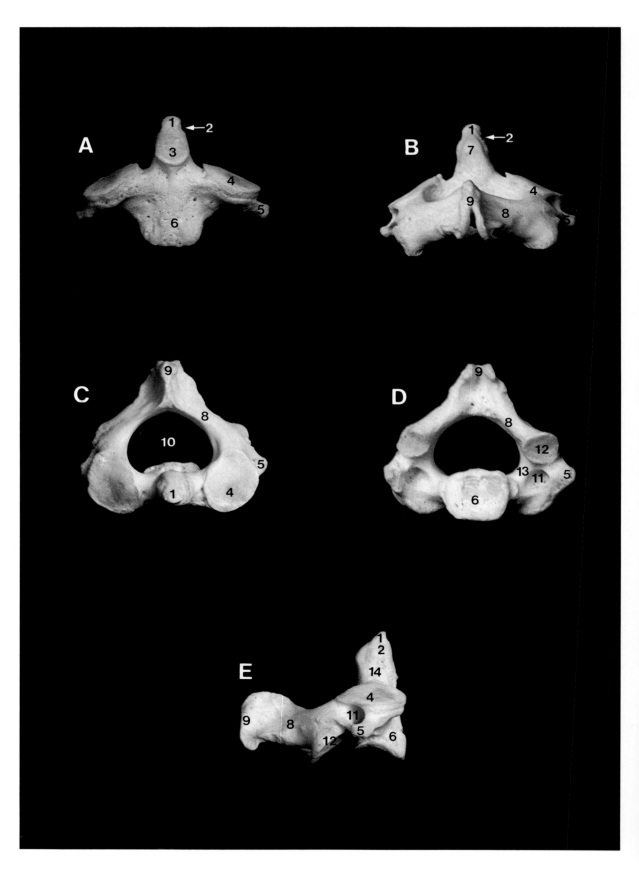

THE AXIS (Second Cervical Vertebra)

A From the front
B From behind
C From above
D From below
E From the right
F Articulated with the atlas, from above and behind

  1 Apex of dens
  2 Impression for alar ligament
  3 Anterior articular surface of dens
  4 Superior articular process
  5 Transverse process
  6 Body
  7 Posterior articular surface of dens
  8 Lamina
  9 Bifid spinous process
10 Vertebral foramen
11 Foramen of transverse process
12 Inferior articular process
13 Pedicle
14 Dens
15 Anterior arch of atlas
16 Dens of axis

●   The anterior articular surface of the dens of the axis forms a synovial joint with the facet on the posterior surface of the anterior arch of the atlas.
●   The posterior articular surface of the dens forms a synovial joint (sometimes continuous with the joint cavity of one of the atlanto-occipital joints) with the cartilage-covered anterior surface of the transverse ligament of the atlas.
●   The axis is unique in having the dens (odontoid process) which projects upwards from the body, and represents the body of the atlas.
●   The spinous process is large and often almost rectangular in shape when viewed from the side.

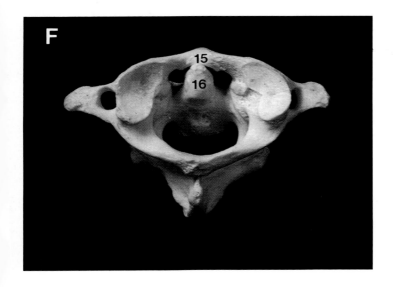

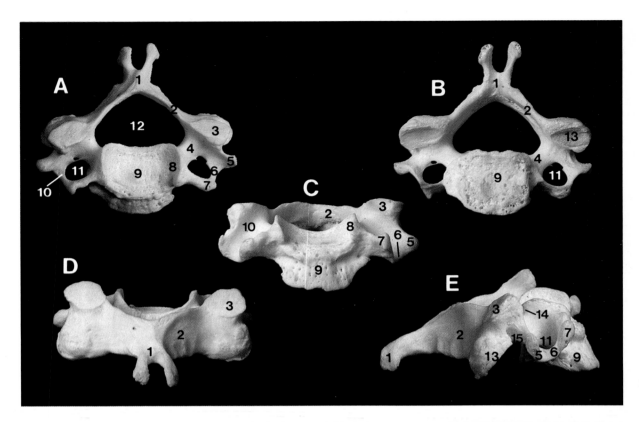

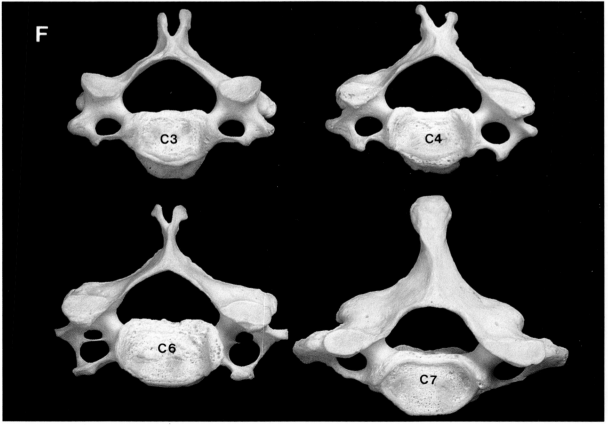

A TYPICAL CERVICAL VERTEBRA (FIFTH)

A From above
B From below
C From the front
D From behind
E From the right

1 Bifid spinous process
2 Lamina
3 Superior articular process
4 Pedicle
5 Posterior tubercle ⎫
6 Costotransverse bar ⎬ of transverse process
7 Anterior tubercle ⎭
8 Uncus (posterolateral lip) of body
9 Body
10 Groove for spinal nerve (ventral ramus)
11 Foramen of transverse process
12 Vertebral foramen
13 Inferior articular process
14 Superior ⎫ vertebral notch
15 Inferior ⎭

● The vertebral arch is formed by the two pedicles and the two laminae

● The vertebral foramen is the space between the arch and the body. When vertebrae are articulated to form a column, the serial vertebral foramina constitute the vertebral canal.

● The intervertebral foramen is the space between adjacent pedicles when vertebrae are articulated (see page 83).

● The spinous process is commonly called the spine.

● The typical cervical vertebrae (3–6) have superior articular processes that face backwards and upwards, an uncus (posterolateral lip) at each side of the upper surface of the body, a triangular vertebral foramen, and a bifid spinous process.

● The seventh cervical vertebra (vertebra prominens) has a spinous process that ends in a single tubercle.

● The costal element of a cervical vertebra is represented by the anterior root of the transverse process, the anterior tubercle, the costotransverse bar and the anterior part of the posterior tubercle.

OTHER CERVICAL VERTEBRAE

F Third, fourth, sixth and seventh vertebrae, from above and numbered C3, C4, C6 and C7 respectively

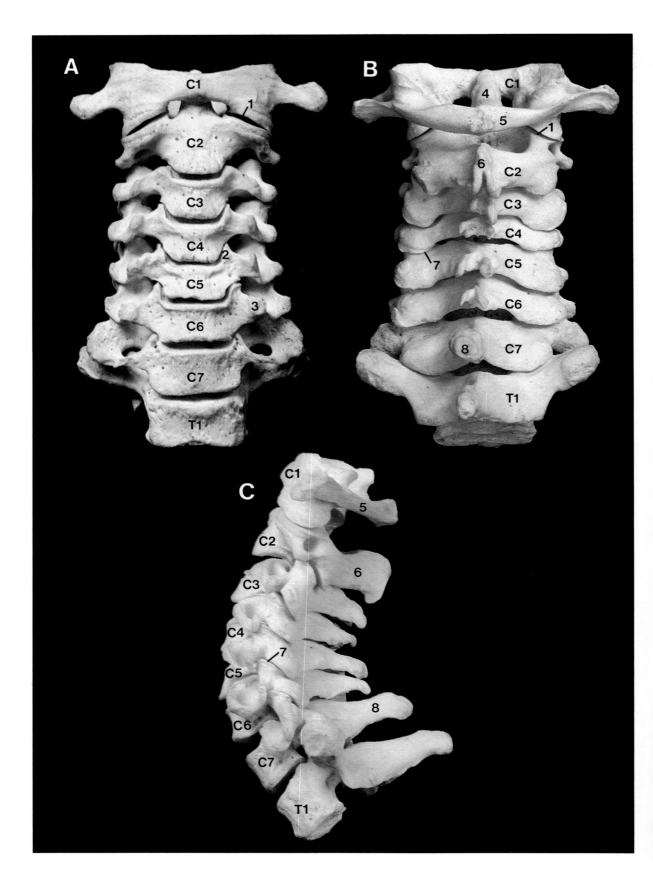

82

CERVICAL VERTEBRAE

Articulated (but without intervertebral discs) and numbered (C1–C7), and with the first thoracic vertebra (T1)

A From the front
B From behind
C From the left

1 Lateral atlanto-axial joint
2 Uncus of fifth cervical vertebra
3 Carotid tubercle of sixth cervical vertebra
4 Dens of axis
5 Posterior arch of atlas
6 Spinous process of axis
7 Zygapophysial joint
8 Spinous process of seventh cervical vertebra

● The cervical curvature of the vertebral column has an anterior convexity (like the lumbar curvature; the thoracic and sacral curvatures are *concave* anteriorly).

● The spinous process of the seventh cervical vertebra projects farther backwards than other cervical spines, and is the highest palpable spine in the median furrow at the back of the neck.

Intervertebral foramen

D Fourth and fifth cervical vertebrae articulated, from the left and slightly from the front

 9 Body
10 Uncus
11 Pedicle
12 Zygapophysial joint between adjacent inferior and superior articular facets
13 Intervertebral foramen
14 Posterior tubercle ⎫
15 Costotransverse bar ⎬ of transverse process
16 Anterior tubercle ⎭

● The intervertebral foramen is bounded above and below by the pedicles of adjacent vertebrae, in front by the vertebral body and intervertebral disc, and behind by the zygapophysial joint.

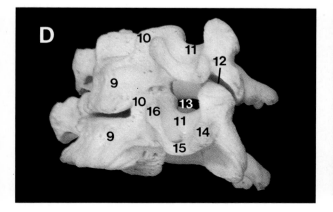

THE FIRST THORACIC VERTEBRA

E From above
F From the left

17 Spinous process
18 Lamina
19 Superior articular process
20 Transverse process
21 Pedicle
22 Uncus of body
23 Body
24 Vertebral foramen
25 Superior vertebral notch
26 Costal facet of transverse process
27 Inferior articular process
28 Inferior vertebral notch
29 Inferior ⎫
30 Superior ⎬ costal facet of body

● Typical thoracic vertebrae (2–9) are characterised by upper and lower articular facets (demifacets) on the sides of the bodies, an articular facet on the front of each transverse process, a round vertebral foramen, a spinous process that points downwards and backwards, and superior articular processes that are vertical, flat and face backwards and laterally.

● The first thoracic vertebra differs from a typical thoracic vertebra in having an uncus on each side of the upper surface of the body and a triangular vertebral foramen (features like typical cervical vertebrae), and a complete (round) superior articular facet (instead of a demifacet) on each side of the body.

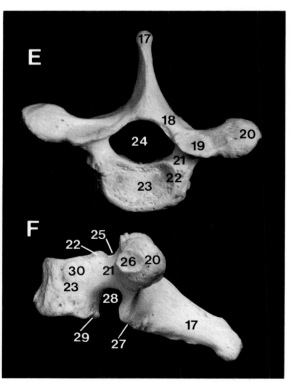

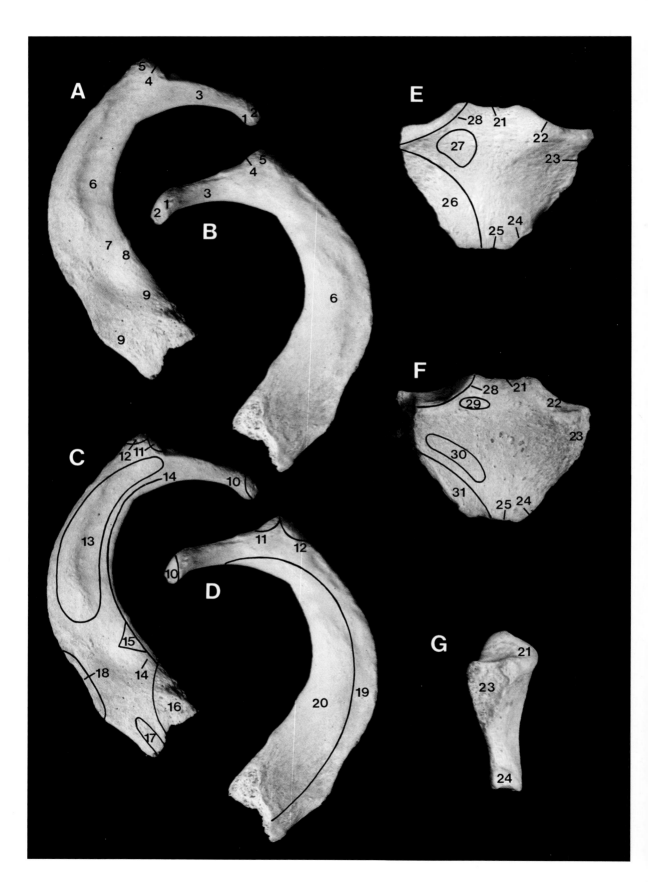

Other Bones

THE FIRST RIB, right

A **From above**
B **From below**
C **From above. Attachments**
D **From below. Attachments**

1 Head
2 Articular surface of head
3 Neck
4 Articular surface of tubercle
5 Tubercle
6 Body
7 Groove for subclavian artery
8 Scalene tubercle
9 Groove for subclavian vein
10 Capsule of joint of head
11 Capsule of costotransverse joint
12 Lateral costotransverse ligament
13 Scalenus medius
14 Suprapleural membrane
15 Scalenus anterior
16 Costoclavicular ligament
17 Subclavius
18 Serratus anterior
19 Intercostal muscles
20 Area covered by pleura

THE MANUBRIUM OF THE STERNUM

E **From the front, with attachments**
F **From behind, with attachments**
G **From the right**

21 Jugular notch
22 Clavicular notch
23 Notch for first costal cartilage
24 Notch for upper part of second costal cartilage
25 Surface for manubriosternal joint
26 Pectoralis major
27 Sternocleidomastoid
28 Capsule of sternoclavicular joint
29 Sternohyoid
30 Sternothyroid
31 Area covered by pleura

H **Articulation of the left first rib with the first thoracic vertebra, from above**

32 Transverse process and costal facet
33 Tubercle and articular facet
34 Head and articular surface
35 Costal facet of body

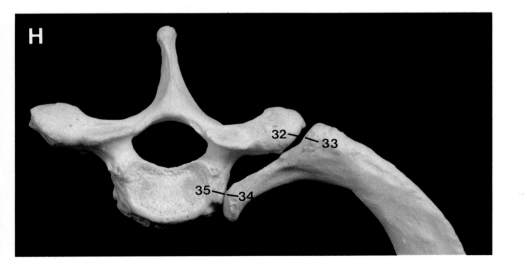

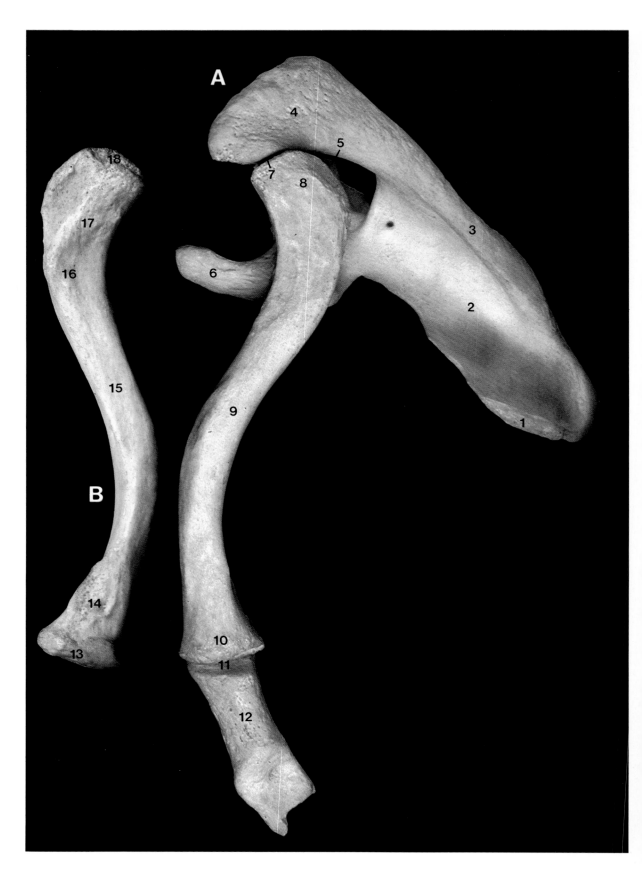

THE CLAVICLE AND SCAPULA, right

A From above, articulated, and with the manubrium of the sternum
B The clavicle, from below

 1 Superior angle
 2 Supraspinous fossa
 3 Spine
 4 Acromion ⎱ of scapula
 5 Upper margin of glenoid cavity
 6 Coracoid process
 7 Acromioclavicular joint
 8 Acromial end
 9 Body ⎱ of clavicle
10 Sternal end
11 Sternoclavicular joint
12 Manubrium of sternum
13 Sternal articular surface
14 Impression for costoclavicular ligament
15 Groove for subclavius muscle
16 Conoid tubercle
17 Trapezoid line
18 Acromial articular surface

● The main features of the clavicle are:
 the bulbous medial (sternal) end
 the flattened lateral (acromial) end
 the groove for the subclavius muscle on the inferior surface

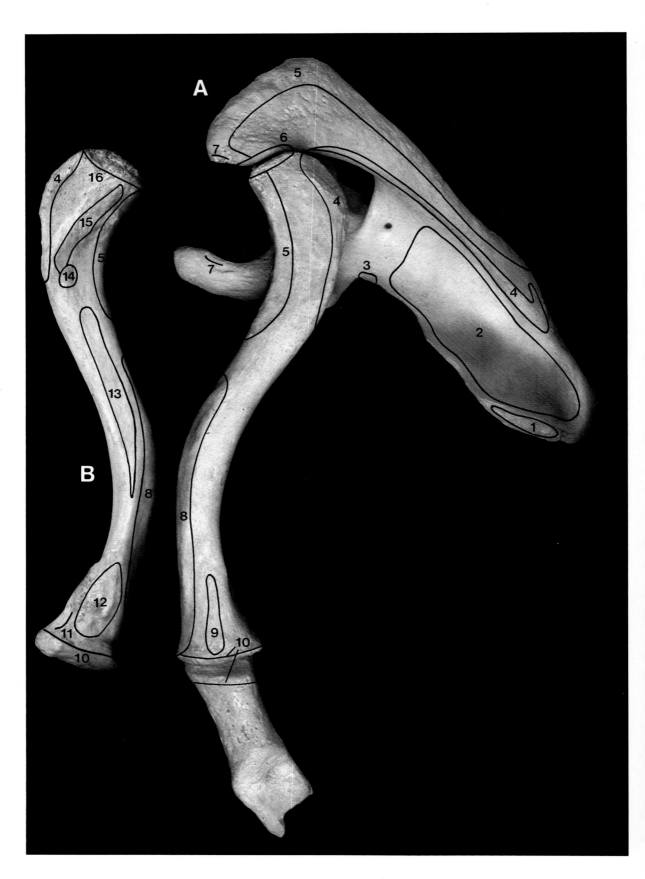

THE CLAVICLE AND SCAPULA

A From above, articulated, and with the manubrium of the sternum. Attachments
B The clavicle, from below. Attachments

  1 Levator scapulae
  2 Supraspinatus
  3 Inferior belly of omohyoid
  4 Trapezius
  5 Deltoid
  6 Capsule of acromioclavicular joint
  7 Coraco-acromial ligament
  8 Pectoralis major
  9 Sternocleidomastoid
10 Capsule of sternoclavicular joint
11 Sternohyoid
12 Costoclavicular ligament
13 Subclavius
14 Conoid ligament ⎱ coracoclavicular
15 Trapezoid ligament ⎰ ligament
16 Capsule of acromioclavicular joint

THE THORACIC INLET

C An articulated skeleton, from the front

17 Seventh cervical vertebra
18 First thoracic vertebra
19 Head ⎫
20 Neck ⎪ of first rib
21 Tubercle ⎬
22 Body ⎭
23 First costal cartilage
24 Sternal end of clavicle
25 Jugular notch of manubrium of sternum

● The thoracic inlet is bounded by the first thoracic vertebra, first ribs and costal cartilages and the manubrium of the sternum.

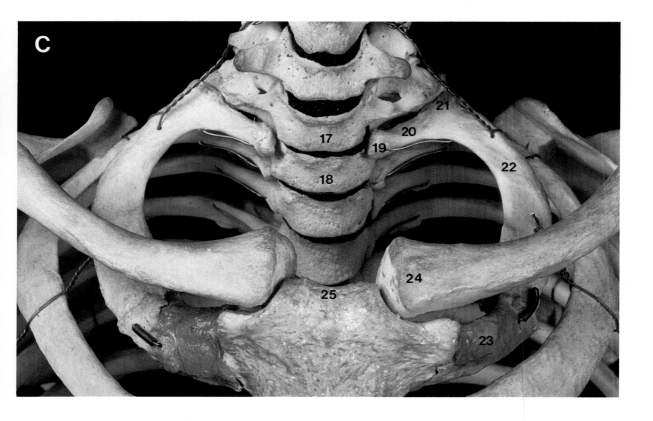

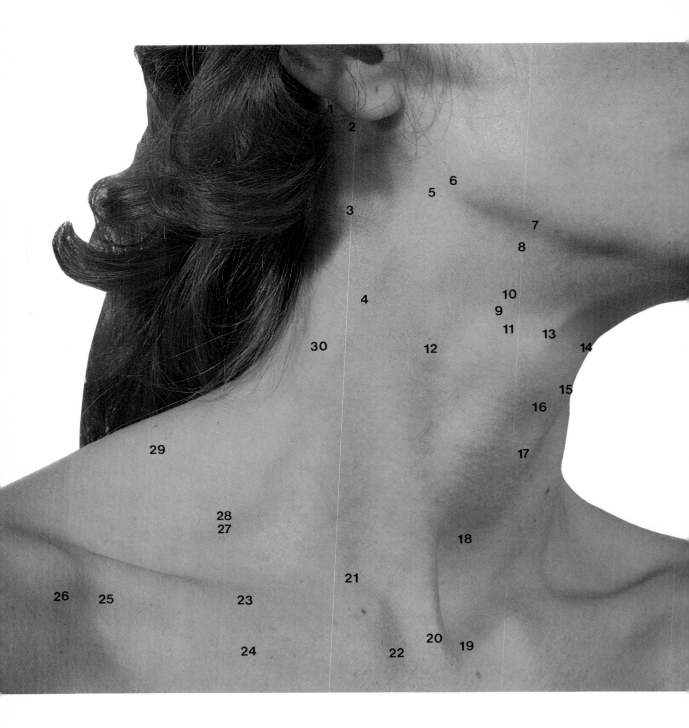

The Neck

Surface markings

Some surface markings on the front and right side of the neck (*For surface markings on the face see page 110*)

1 Mastoid process
2 Tip of transverse process of atlas
3 Sternocleidomastoid
4 External jugular vein
5 Lowest part of parotid gland
6 Angle of mandible
7 Anterior border of masseter and facial artery
8 Submandibular gland
9 Tip of greater horn of hyoid bone
10 Hypoglossal nerve
11 Internal laryngeal nerve
12 Bifurcation of common carotid artery
13 Anterior jugular vein
14 Body of hyoid bone
15 Laryngeal prominence
16 Vocal fold
17 Arch of cricoid cartilage
18 Isthmus of thyroid gland
19 Jugular notch and trachea
20 Sternal head } of sternocleidomastoid
21 Clavicular head
22 Sternoclavicular joint and union of internal jugular and subclavian veins to form brachiocephalic vein
23 Clavicle
24 Pectoralis major
25 Infraclavicular fossa and cephalic vein
26 Deltoid
27 Inferior belly of omohyoid
28 Upper trunk of brachial plexus
29 Trapezius and entry of accessory nerve
30 Accessory nerve emerging from sternocleidomastoid

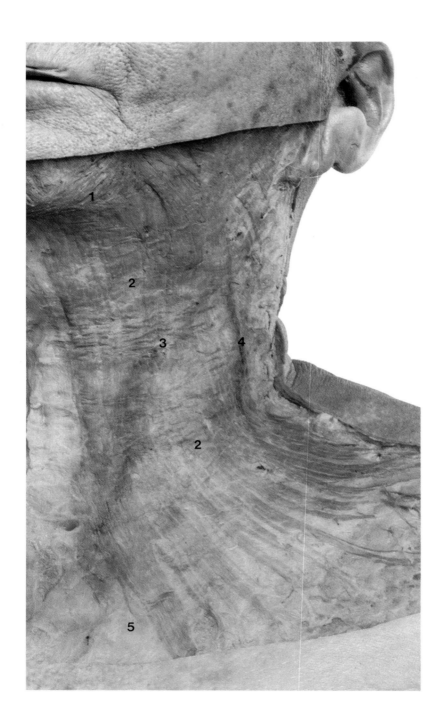

THE NECK

Superficial dissection I

The left platysma, from the front and the left

1 Lower border of body of mandible
2 Platysma
3 Anterior jugular vein
4 External jugular vein
5 Clavicle

● The supraclavicular nerves lie deep to platysma.

● The motor nerve supply of platysma is the cervical branch of the facial nerve.

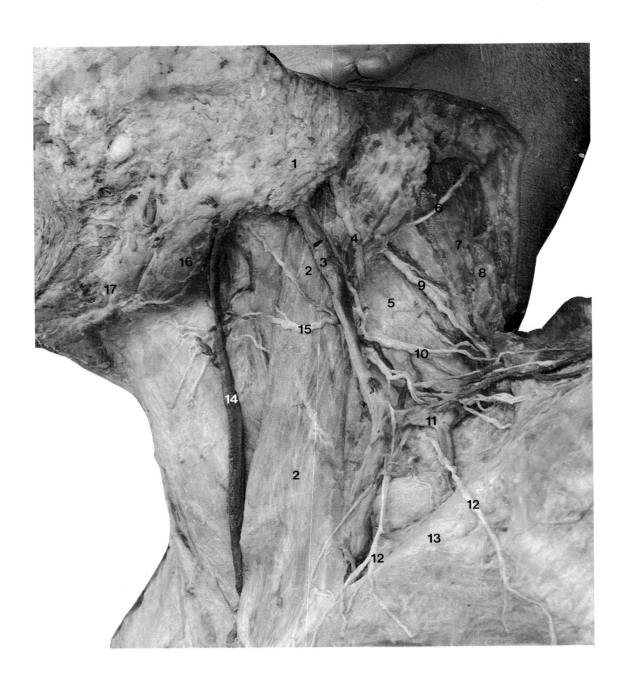

THE NECK

Superficial dissection II

The left sternocleidomastoid and related structures
(after removal of platysma and most of the investing layer of deep cervical fascia)

1 Parotid gland
2 Sternocleidomastoid
3 External jugular vein
4 Great auricular nerve
5 Prevertebral fascia overlying levator scapulae
6 Lesser occipital nerve
7 Splenius capitis
8 Trapezius
9 Accessory nerve
10 Cervical nerves to trapezius
11 Superficial cervical vein
12 Supraclavicular nerves
13 Clavicle
14 Anterior jugular vein
15 Transverse cervical nerve
16 Submandibular gland
17 Lower border of mandible

● The motor nerve supply of sternocleidomastoid is the accessory nerve. The cervical branches to the muscle are afferent.

● The nerve commonly known in English as the accessory nerve (or spinal part of the accessory nerve) is in official anatomical nomenclature the ramus externus of the truncus nervi accessorii. The cells of origin are in the anterior horn of the upper five or six cervical segments of the spinal cord, and the fibres supply sternocleidomastoid and trapezius. (The cranial part of the accessory nerve is derived from the nucleus ambiguus in the medulla oblongata and joins the vagus nerve to supply muscles of the soft palate and larynx.)

● The deep cervical fascia consists of:
the investing layer
the prevertebral layer
the pretracheal layer
the carotid sheath
● The investing layer forms the roof of the posterior triangle, splits to enclose the sternocleidomastoid and trapezius, and forms capsules for the parotid and submandibular glands.
● The prevertebral layer forms the floor of the posterior triangle, lying in front of the vertebral column and prevertebral muscles.
● The pretracheal layer forms a sheath for the thyroid gland.
● The carotid sheath is formed by condensations of the prevertebral and pretracheal layers enclosing the internal jugular vein, common and internal carotid arteries, the vagus nerve, and the ansa cervicalis with its superior and inferior roots. Near the base of the skull the glossopharyngeal and hypoglossal nerves pass through the sheath.

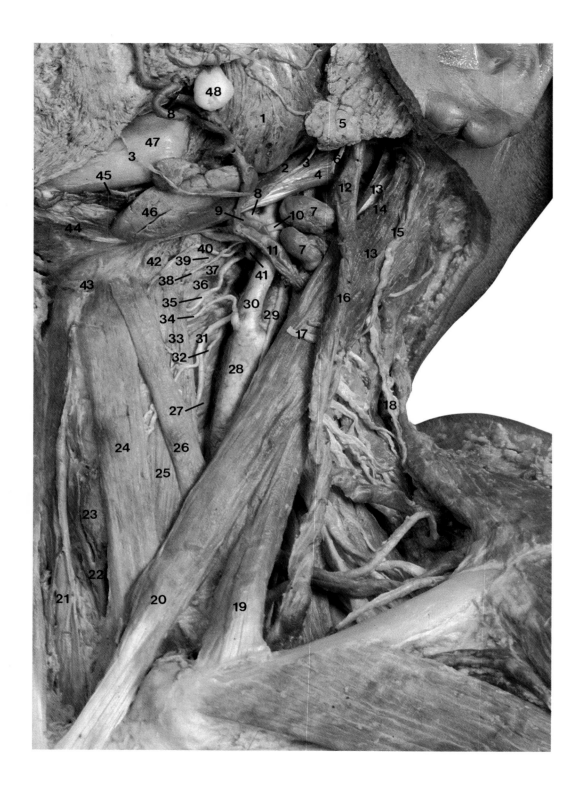

THE NECK

Superficial dissection III

The left anterior triangle *(Details of the posterior triangle in this specimen are given on the next page)*

1 Masseter
2 Stylohyoid
3 Marginal mandibular branch of facial nerve
4 Posterior belly of digastric
5 Parotid gland
6 Cervical branch of facial nerve
7 Jugulodigastric lymph nodes
8 Facial artery
9 Lingual vein
10 Hypoglossal nerve
11 Facial vein
12 Posterior branch of retromandibular vein
13 Sternocleidomastoid
14 Posterior auricular vein
15 Great auricular nerve
16 External jugular vein
17 Transverse cervical nerve
18 Accessory nerve
19 Clavicular head } of sternocleidomastoid
20 Sternal head
21 Anterior jugular vein
22 Inferior thyroid vein
23 Thyroid gland
24 Sternohyoid
25 Sternothyroid
26 Superior belly of omohyoid
27 Inferior constrictor of pharynx
28 Common carotid artery
29 Internal carotid artery and superior root of ansa cervicalis
30 External carotid artery
31 Superior thyroid artery
32 External laryngeal nerve
33 Thyrohyoid
34 Superior laryngeal artery
35 Internal laryngeal nerve
36 Thyrohyoid membrane
37 Greater horn of hyoid bone
38 Nerve to thyrohyoid
39 Hyoglossus
40 Suprahyoid artery
41 Lingual artery
42 Mylohyoid
43 Body of hyoid bone
44 Anterior belly of digastric
45 Submental artery and vein
46 Submandibular gland
47 Body of mandible
48 Buccal fat pad

● Triangles of the neck:
  Anterior triangle, subdivided into
    Submental triangle
    Digastric triangle
    Muscular triangle
    Carotid triangle
  Posterior triangle

● The anterior triangle is bounded by the mandible, the midline and sternocleidomastoid.

● The posterior triangle is bounded by sternocleidomastoid, trapezius and the middle third of the clavicle.

● Anterior triangle
  Boundaries: sternocleidomastoid, lower border of the mandible and the midline. It is subdivided into the submental, digastric, muscular and carotid triangles.

● Submental triangle
  Boundaries: anterior belly of digastric, body of the hyoid bone and the midline.
  Floor: mylohyoid.
  Contents: anterior jugular vein and submental lymph nodes.

● Digastric triangle
  Boundaries: the two bellies of digastric and the lower border of the mandible.
  Floor: mylohyoid, hyoglossus, middle constrictor.
  Contents: submandibular gland and lymph nodes, and the lower part of the parotid gland posteriorly; facial artery and vein and submental vessels, and the carotid sheath posteriorly; hypoglossal nerve, mylohyoid nerve and vessels, stylopharyngeus and the glossopharyngeal nerve.

● Muscular triangle
  Boundaries: sternocleidomastoid, superior belly of omohyoid and the midline.
  Floor: sternothyroid, sternohyoid.
  Contents (beneath the floor): thyroid gland, larynx, trachea, oesophagus.

● Carotid triangle
  Boundaries: sternocleidomastoid, posterior belly of digastric and superior belly of omohyoid.
  Floor: thyrohyoid, hyoglossus, middle and inferior constrictors.
  Contents: bifurcation of the common carotid artery; superior thyroid, lingual, facial, occipital and ascending pharyngeal branches of the external carotid artery; hypoglossal nerve and its two branches – nerve to thyrohyoid and superior root of ansa cervicalis; internal and external laryngeal nerves.

● For notes on the submandibular gland see page 141.

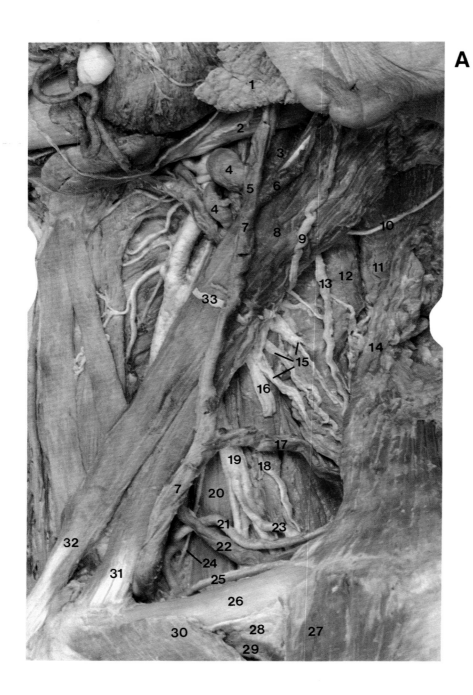

THE NECK

Superficial dissection IV

The left posterior triangle *(Details of the anterior triangle in A are given on the previous page)*

A From the left
B The upper part of the triangle, from behind

1 Parotid gland
2 Posterior belly of digastric
3 Internal jugular vein
4 Jugulodigastric lymph nodes
5 Posterior branch of retromandibular vein
6 Posterior auricular vein
7 External jugular vein
8 Sternocleidomastoid
9 Great auricular nerve
10 Lesser occipital nerve
11 Splenius capitis
12 Levator scapulae
13 Accessory nerve
14 Trapezius
15 Cervical nerves to trapezius
16 Supraclavicular nerve
17 Superficial cervical vein
18 Dorsal scapular nerve
19 Upper trunk of brachial plexus
20 Scalenus anterior
21 Superficial cervical artery
22 Inferior belly of omohyoid
23 Suprascapular nerve
24 Phrenic nerve
25 Suprascapular artery
26 Clavicle
27 Deltoid
28 Clavipectoral fascia
29 Cephalic vein
30 Pectoralis major
31 Clavicular head ⎱
32 Sternal head   ⎰ of sternocleidomastoid
33 Transverse cervical nerve
34 Occipital vein
35 Occipital belly of occipitofrontalis
36 Greater occipital nerve
37 Occipital artery
38 Semispinalis capitis
39 Third occipital nerve

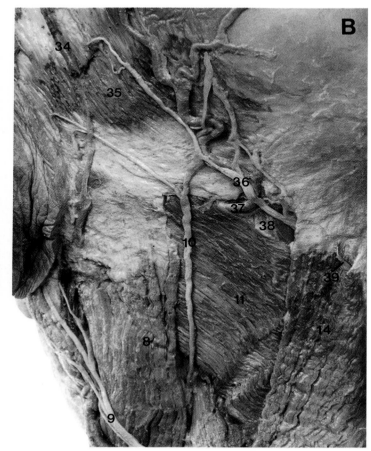

● Posterior triangle
  Boundaries: sternocleidomastoid, trapezius and the middle third of the clavicle.
  Floor: the prevertebral layer of the deep cervical fascia.
  Contents: arteries – occipital, superficial cervical, suprascapular, subclavian.
  veins – external jugular, superficial cervical, suprascapular.
  nerves – branches of the cervical plexus (great auricular, lesser occipital, transverse cervical, supraclavicular and muscular).
  trunks of the brachial plexus, the branches of the upper trunk (nerve to subclavius and suprascapular) and the dorsal scapular nerve (from the uppermost root of the plexus).
  accessory nerve (embedded in the investing layer of deep cervical fascia that forms the roof of the triangle).
  muscle – inferior belly of omohyoid.
  lymph nodes.

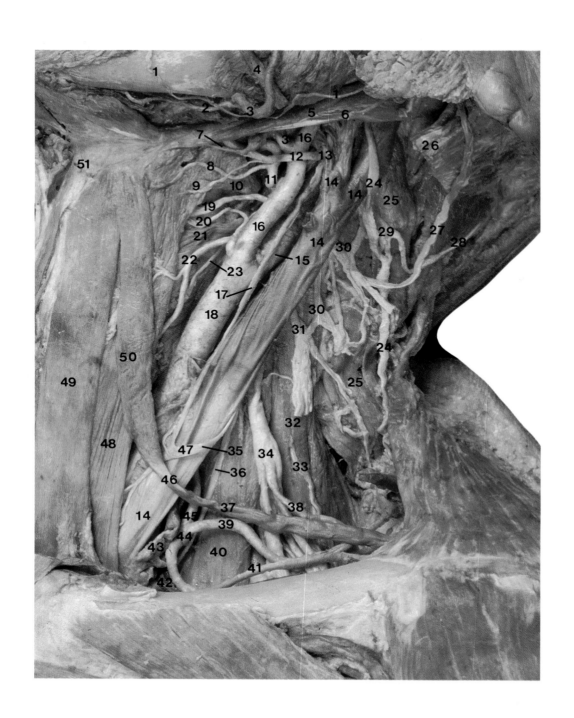

THE NECK

Deep dissection I

Great vessels and nerves of the left side *(with most of sternocleidomastoid and the submandibular gland removed)*

1 Marginal mandibular branch of facial nerve
2 Submental artery
3 Facial artery
4 Facial vein
5 Stylohyoid
6 Posterior belly of digastric
7 Vena comitans of hypoglossal nerve
8 Suprahyoid artery and hyoglossus
9 Thyrohyoid and nerve
10 Greater horn of hyoid bone
11 Lingual artery
12 Hypoglossal nerve
13 Lingual vein
14 Internal jugular vein (double at upper end)
15 Internal carotid artery and carotid sinus
16 External carotid artery
17 Superior root of ansa cervicalis
18 Common carotid artery
19 Internal laryngeal nerve and thyrohyoid membrane
20 Superior laryngeal artery
21 Inferior constrictor of pharynx
22 Superior thyroid artery
23 External laryngeal nerve
24 Accessory nerve
25 Levator scapulae
26 Sternocleidomastoid
27 Great auricular nerve
28 Lesser occipital nerve
29 Second ⎫
30 Third ⎬ cervical nerve ventral rami
31 Fourth ⎭
32 Scalenus medius
33 Dorsal scapular nerve
34 Upper trunk of brachial plexus
35 Inferior root of ansa cervicalis
36 Phrenic nerve
37 Inferior belly of omohyoid
38 Suprascapular nerve
39 Superficial cervical artery
40 Scalenus anterior
41 Suprascapular artery
42 Subclavian vein
43 Thoracic duct
44 Thyrocervical trunk
45 Inferior thyroid artery
46 Omohyoid tendon
47 Ansa cervicalis
48 Sternothyroid
49 Sternohyoid
50 Superior belly of omohyoid
51 Hyoid bone

● The hypoglossal nerve passes forwards *above* the tip of the greater horn of the hyoid bone; the internal laryngeal nerve passes downwards and forwards *below* the tip of the greater horn (see also page 90).

● The common carotid artery divides into the external and internal carotids at about the level of the upper border of the thyroid cartilage (fourth cervical vertebra).

● The external carotid artery can be distinguished readily from the internal carotid as it gives off a number of branches; the internal carotid gives no branches in the neck.

● The carotid sinus is a baroreceptor (pressure receptor) at the commencement of the internal carotid artery (within its wall).

● The carotid body is a chemoreceptor behind or between the bifurcation of the common carotid artery. An oval body a few millimeters long, it contains glomus cells within a connective tissue capsule.

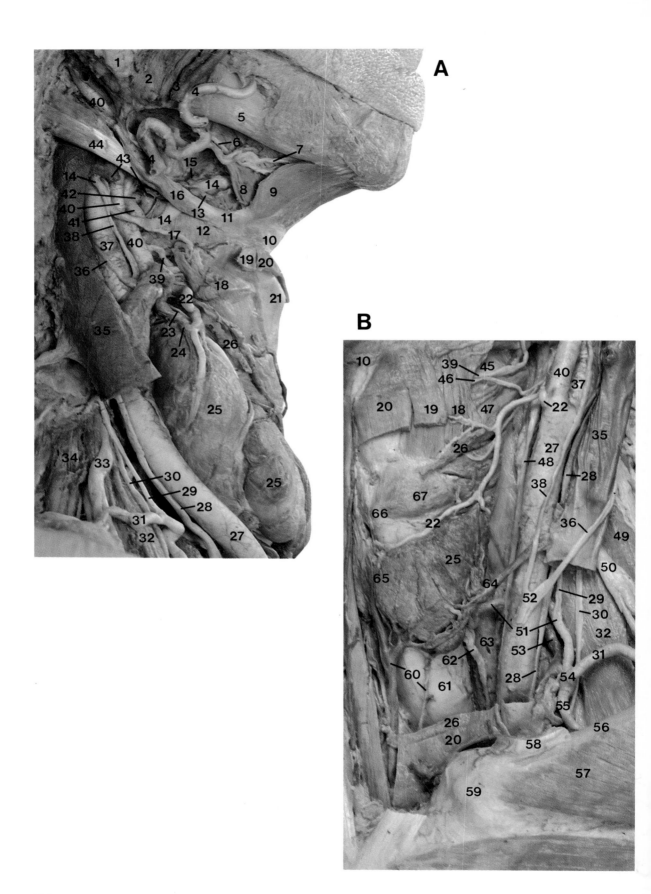

THE NECK

Deep dissection II

The great vessels and the thyroid gland

A From the right
B From the front and left

1 Parotid gland
2 Masseter
3 Facial vein
4 Facial artery
5 Body of mandible
6 Nerve to mylohyoid
7 Submental artery
8 Mylohyoid
9 Anterior belly of digastric
10 Body of hyoid bone
11 Digastric tendon
12 Hyoglossus
13 Vena comitans of hypoglossal nerve
14 Hypoglossal nerve
15 A tributary of 13
16 Stylohyoid
17 Nerve to thyrohyoid
18 Thyrohyoid
19 Superior belly of omohyoid
20 Sternohyoid
21 Laryngeal prominence
22 Superior thyroid artery
23 External laryngeal nerve
24 Superior thyroid vein
25 Lateral lobe of thyroid gland
26 Sternothyroid
27 Common carotid artery
28 Vagus nerve
29 Ascending cervical artery
30 Phrenic nerve
31 Superficial cervical artery
32 Scalenus anterior
33 Ventral ramus of fifth cervical nerve
34 Scalenus medius
35 Internal jugular vein
36 Inferior root of ansa cervicalis
37 Internal carotid artery
38 Superior root of ansa cervicalis
39 Internal laryngeal nerve
40 External carotid artery
41 Linguofacial trunk
42 Lingual artery
43 Lingual vein
44 Posterior belly of digastric
45 Thyrohyoid membrane
46 Superior laryngeal artery
47 Inferior constrictor of pharynx
48 Sympathetic trunk
49 Scalenus medius
50 Upper trunk of brachial plexus
51 Inferior thyroid artery
52 Ansa cervicalis
53 Thoracic duct
54 Thyrocervical trunk
55 Suprascapular artery
56 Clavicle
57 Pectoralis major
58 Sternocleidomastoid
59 Capsule of sternoclavicular joint
60 Inferior thyroid veins
61 Trachea
62 Recurrent laryngeal nerve
63 Oesophagus
64 Middle thyroid vein
65 Isthmus of thyroid gland
66 Arch of cricoid cartilage
67 Cricothyroid

● The thyroid gland is enclosed in a sheath derived from the pretracheal fascia, which attaches it to the larynx (hence it moves with the larynx during swallowing).
● It extends from the level of C5 to T1 vertebra.
● The isthmus of the gland overlies tracheal rings 2 and 3, with an anastomosis between the superior thyroid arteries of each side along the upper border, and a variable number of veins passing down from the lower border.
● Important relations of the lateral lobes include:
    laterally – sternothyroid (which limits upward extension of the gland), sternohyoid, omohyoid and sternocleido-mastoid.
    medially – the larynx and trachea, pharynx and oesophagus, cricothyroid, the inferior constrictor of the pharynx, the external and recurrent laryngeal nerves.
    posterolaterally – the common carotid artery within the carotid sheath, the parathyroid glands, the inferior thyroid artery, the thoracic duct (on the left).
● The external laryngeal nerve lies just behind the superior thyroid artery as the artery approaches the upper pole of the lateral lobe. Ligation of the artery during thyroidectomy is carried out at the tip of the pole, to avoid damaging the nerve.
● The recurrent laryngeal nerve (which enters the larynx by passing under the lower border of the inferior constrictor of the pharynx, immediately posterior to the cricothyroid joint) lies either anterior or posterior to the inferior thyroid artery as the artery arches medially behind the lower part of the lateral lobe. Ligation of the artery is carried out well away from the gland to avoid damaging the nerve.

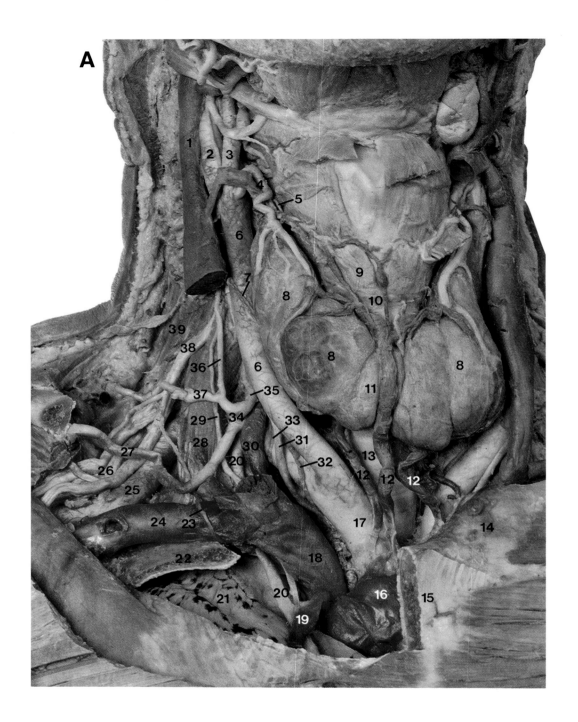

A

THE NECK

Deep dissection III

The thyroid gland and the root of the neck

A The thyroid gland and the root of the neck on the right side *(with partial removal of the right clavicle, first rib and manubrium of the sternum)*

1 Internal jugular vein
2 Internal carotid artery
3 External carotid artery
4 Superior thyroid artery and vein
5 External laryngeal nerve
6 Common carotid artery
7 Middle thyroid vein
8 Lateral lobe of thyroid gland
9 Cricothyroid
10 Arch of cricoid cartilage
11 Isthmus of thyroid gland
12 Inferior thyroid veins
13 Trachea
14 Capsule of sternoclavicular joint
15 Manubrium of sternum
16 Left brachiocephalic vein
17 Brachiocephalic artery
18 Right brachiocephalic vein
19 Internal thoracic vein
20 Internal thoracic artery
21 Lung
22 First rib
23 Accessory phrenic nerve
24 Subclavian vein
25 Subclavian artery
26 Brachial plexus
27 Suprascapular artery
28 Scalenus anterior
29 Phrenic nerve
30 Vertebral vein

31 Vagus nerve
32 Jugular lymphatic trunk
33 Ansa subclavia
34 Thyrocervical trunk
35 Inferior thyroid artery
36 Ascending cervical artery
37 Superficial cervical artery
38 Ventral ramus of fifth cervical nerve
39 Scalenus medius

B An isolated thyroid gland, from behind, with parathyroid glands

40 Superior thyroid artery and vein
41 Right superior parathyroid gland
42 Posterior border of right lateral lobe
43 Branches of inferior thyroid artery
44 Right inferior parathyroid gland
45 Inferior thyroid veins
46 Isthmus
47 Left superior parathyroid gland

● A pyramidal lobe of the thyroid gland is often present; it passes from the upper part of the isthmus or adjoining part of a lateral lobe (usually the left) towards the hyoid bone. A fibrous or fibromuscular band may connect the isthmus or the pyramidal lobe to the hyoid bone; if muscular it constitutes the levator of the thyroid gland (see page 139).

● The typical number of parathyroid glands is four (in 90% of subjects) but there may be more or less; in B there are only three.
● They usually lie between the posterior surface of the lateral lobes of the thyroid gland and the thin capsule of the gland (which is inside the fascial sheath).
● The blood supply of both the superior and inferior parathyroid glands is mainly from the *inferior* thyroid artery.

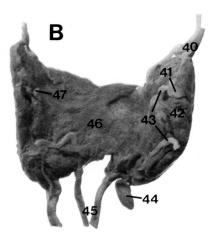

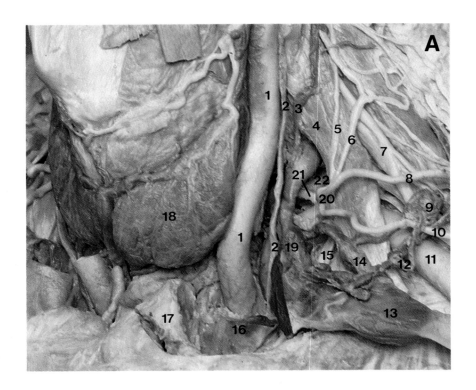

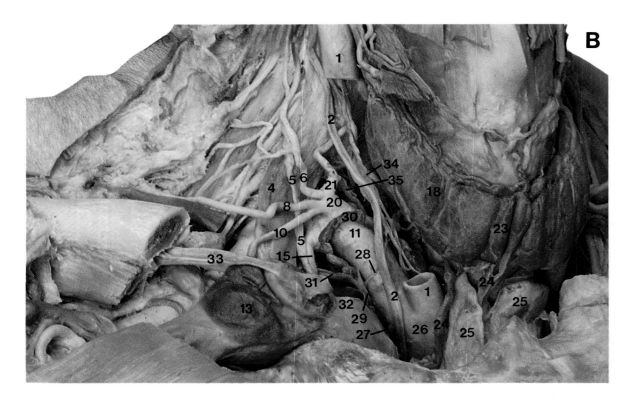

THE NECK

Deep dissection IV

The thyroid gland, root of the neck, thoracic duct, right lymphatic duct and the thymus

A The left side, from the front and the left
B The right side, from the front and the right

1 Common carotid artery
2 Vagus nerve
3 Ascending cervical vein
4 Scalenus anterior
5 Phrenic nerve
6 Ascending cervical artery
7 Upper trunk of brachial plexus
8 Superficial cervical artery
9 A lower deep cervical lymph node
10 Suprascapular artery
11 Subclavian artery
12 A subclavian lymphatic trunk
13 Subclavian vein
14 Thoracic duct
15 Internal thoracic artery
16 Brachiocephalic vein
17 Disc of sternoclavicular joint
18 Lateral lobe of thyroid gland
19 Vertebral vein
20 Thyrocervical trunk
21 Inferior thyroid artery
22 Vertebral artery
23 Isthmus of thyroid gland
24 Inferior thyroid veins
25 Lobes of persistent thymus gland
26 Brachiocephalic artery
27 Recurrent laryngeal nerve
28 Ansa subclavia
29 Right lymphatic duct
30 Mediastinal lymphatic trunk
31 Subclavian lymphatic trunk
32 Cut end of internal jugular vein
33 Suprascapular vein
34 Sympathetic trunk and middle cervical ganglion
35 Tracheal branch of inferior thyroid artery

● In A, the inferior thyroid artery arises directly from the subclavian artery instead of the thyrocervical trunk, and the ascending cervical artery which is normally a branch of the inferior thyroid comes from the thyrocervical trunk in place of the inferior thyroid. Because of its unusual origin the inferior thyroid artery has passed behind the vertebral vein instead of in front of it.

● The sympathetic nervous system in the neck consists of the sympathetic trunk with the superior, middle and inferior cervical sympathetic ganglia and their branches.

● The rather elongated superior cervical ganglion lies at the level of the second and third cervical vertebrae between longuş capitis (behind) and the internal carotid artery within the carotid sheath (in front). It gives off from its upper end the internal carotid nerve, which constitutes the cephalic part of the sympathetic nervous system and enters the cranial cavity with the internal carotid artery. Other branches include grey rami communicantes to the upper four cervical nerves, a cardiac branch and branches to cervical viscera and vessels and the carotid body.

● The middle cervical ganglion (the smallest of the three) is at the level of the sixth cervical vertebra, usually in front of the inferior thyroid artery and always in front of the vertebral artery. It gives grey rami communicantes to the fifth and sixth cervical nerves, forms the ansa subclavia, and gives a cardiac branch and branches to cervical viscera and vessels.

● The inferior cervical ganglion lies in front of the neck of the first rib and behind the vertebral artery; it is frequently fused with the first thoracic sympathetic ganglion to form the cervicothoracic (stellate) ganglion. It gives grey rami communicantes to the seventh and eighth cervical nerves (and to the first thoracic nerve if fused), a cardiac branch and branches to adjacent vessels.

● The middle cervical ganglion lies *in front* of the vertebral artery; the inferior cervical ganglion lies *behind* it.

● At the level of the sixth cervical vertebra:
the cricoid cartilage
the larynx continues as the trachea
the pharynx continues as the oesophagus
the middle cervical sympathetic ganglion
the vertebral artery enters the foramen of the transverse process
the inferior thyroid artery arches medially

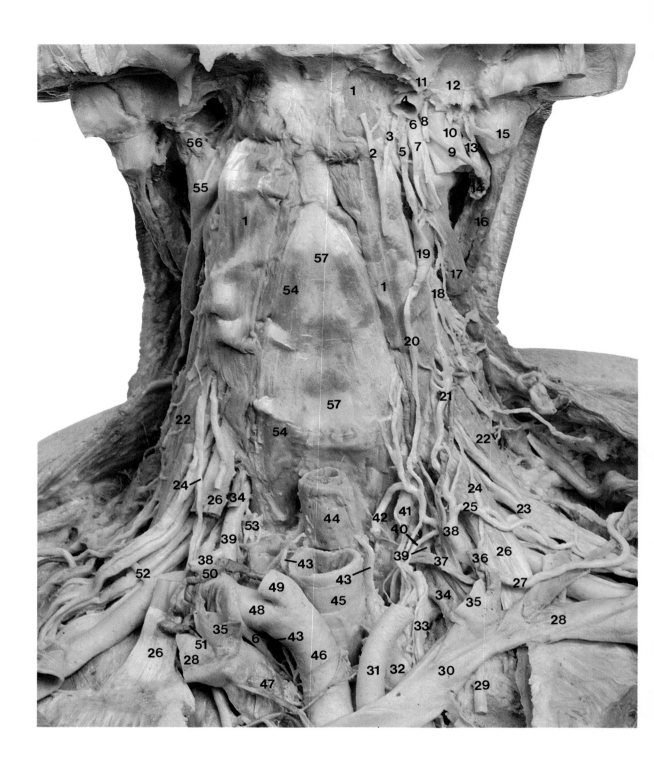

THE NECK

Deep dissection V

The prevertebral muscles (*For the posterior part of the neck see pages 198 –201*)

1 Longus capitis
2 Ascending pharyngeal artery
3 Meningeal branch of ascending pharyngeal artery
4 Internal carotid artery
5 Internal carotid nerve
6 Vagus nerve
7 Inferior vagal ganglion
8 Glossopharyngeal nerve
9 Accessory nerve (spinal root)
10 Internal jugular vein
11 Spine of sphenoid bone
12 Tympanic part of temporal bone
13 Occipital artery
14 Posterior belly of digastric
15 Mastoid process
16 Sternocleidomastoid
17 Levator scapulae
18 Ventral ramus of third cervical nerve
19 Superior cervical ganglion
20 Sympathetic trunk
21 Ascending cervical artery and vein
22 Scalenus medius
23 Upper trunk of brachial plexus
24 Phrenic nerve
25 Superficial cervical artery
26 Scalenus anterior
27 Suprascapular artery
28 Subclavian vein
29 Internal thoracic artery
30 Left brachiocephalic vein
31 Left common carotid artery
32 Left subclavian artery
33 Vagus nerve
34 Vertebral vein
35 Internal jugular vein
36 Jugular lymphatic trunk
37 Thoracic duct
38 Thyrocervical trunk
39 Vertebral artery
40 A large oesophageal branch of inferior thyroid artery
41 Middle cervical ganglion
42 Inferior thyroid artery
43 Recurrent laryngeal nerve
44 Oesophagus
45 Trachea
46 Brachiocephalic artery
47 Right brachiocephalic vein
48 Right subclavian artery
49 Right common carotid artery
50 Mediastinal lymphatic trunk
51 Right lymphatic duct
52 Dorsal scapular artery
53 Inferior cervical ganglion
54 Longus colli
55 Transverse process of atlas
56 Rectus capitis lateralis
57 Anterior longitudinal ligament

● In the lower neck, the thoracic duct lies behind the left margin of the oesophagus and then arches laterally between the carotid sheath (in front) and the vertebral vessels, sympathetic trunk and thyrocervical trunk and its branches (behind) to enter the junction of the internal jugular and subclavian veins.

The Face

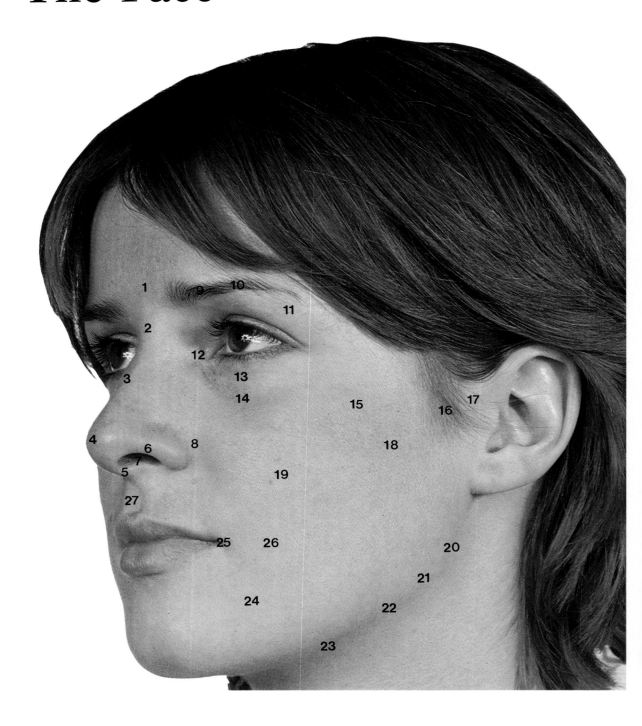

THE FACE

Surface markings

Some surface markings on the front and left side of the face *(For details of the eye see page 118, and of the ear see page 148. For surface markings on the neck see page 90)*

1 Glabella
2 Root ⎫
3 Dorsum ⎪
4 Apex ⎪
5 Septum ⎬ of nose
6 Ala ⎪
7 Anterior naris ⎪
8 Alar groove ⎭
9 Frontal notch and supratrochlear nerve and artery
10 Supra-orbital notch (or foramen), nerve and artery
11 Lateral part of supra-orbital margin
12 Medial palpebral ligament and lacrimal sac
13 Infra-orbital margin
14 Infra-orbital foramen, nerve and vessels
15 Zygomatic arch
16 Head of mandible
17 Auriculotemporal nerve and superficial temporal artery
18 Parotid duct emerging from gland
19 Parotid duct turning medially at anterior border of masseter
20 Angle of mandible
21 Lower border of ramus
22 Anterior border of masseter and facial artery and vein
23 Lower border of body of mandible
24 Mental foramen, nerve and artery
25 Lateral angle of mouth
26 Modiolus
27 Philtrum

● The anterior naris is commonly called the nostril.

● The muscles of the face (including buccinator) and platysma are all supplied by the facial nerve.

● Facial nerve paralysis (Bell's palsy):
  The lower eyelid droops (but *not* the upper lid, which is supplied by the oculomotor nerve), and the cornea may become damaged by dryness because the eye cannot be closed properly
  The angle of the mouth droops, with dribbling of saliva, and it is not possible to 'show the teeth' on the affected side.
  Whistling is not possible, and food collects between the teeth and the cheek (due to paralysis of the buccinator).

● The facial paralysis may be accompanied by the following additional features depending on the site of the damage. If the damage:
  is in the pons (where the facial nerve fibres overlie the abducent nucleus) there may be paralysis of the lateral rectus.
  is in the cerebellopontine angle or internal acoustic meatus where the facial and vestibulocochlear nerves lie close together, there may be deafness.
  involves the nerve to stapedius, there may be hyperacusis (extreme sensitivity to sound) due to loss of the dampening effect on the vibration of the stapes.
  involves the chorda tympani, there may be loss of taste sensation from the anterior two-thirds of the tongue (the unilateral loss of submandibular and sublingual secretion will not be noticed).

● The above notes on facial nerve paralysis refer to 'infranuclear paralysis', i.e. damage to the axons derived from the facial nerve nucleus in the pons.

● Supranuclear paralysis refers to paralysis due to interruption of the pathway from the cerebral cortex to the facial nerve nucleus, i.e. damage to corticonuclear fibres. The axons from the cell bodies of the upper part of the facial nerve nucleus (in the pons) supply the forehead muscle (frontal belly of occipitofrontalis) and receive corticonuclear fibres from the cerebral cortex of both sides, i.e. there are two sources of corticonuclear supply. The lower part of the facial nerve nucleus supplying the lower facial muscles and platysma receives corticonuclear fibres from the opposite cerebral cortex only, i.e. only one source of corticonuclear supply. Therefore unilateral supranuclear lesions (e.g. from haemorrhage in the internal capsule involving corticonuclear fibres) causes paralysis of the lower facial muscles of the opposite (contralateral) side but does not affect movement of the forehead on that side, because the neurons supplying the forehead muscle still have an intact corticonuclear supply from the same (ipsilateral) side.

● The superficial temporal artery can be palpated behind the head of the mandible (where the artery crosses the root of the zygomatic process of the temporal bone).

● The facial artery can be palpated as it passes from the neck on to the face 2.5 cm in front of the angle of the mandible.

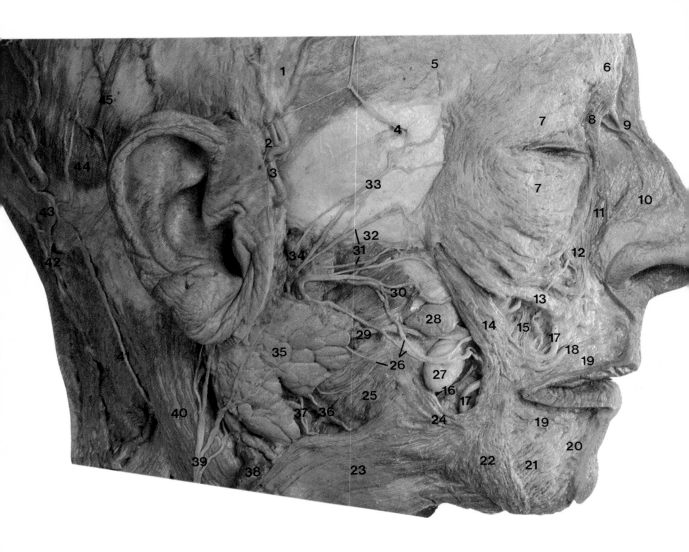

THE FACE

Superficial dissection

The right parotid gland, facial nerve and facial muscles *(with removal of the upper part of the parotid gland)*

1 Temporoparietalis
2 Auriculotemporal nerve
3 Superficial temporal artery
4 Zygomaticotemporal nerve piercing temporalis fascia
5 Epicranial aponeurosis (galea aponeurotica)
6 Frontal belly of occipitofrontalis
7 Orbicularis oculi
8 Depressor supercilii
9 Procerus
10 Nasalis
11 Levator labii superioris alaeque nasi
12 Levator labii superioris
13 Zygomaticus minor
14 Zygomaticus major
15 Levator anguli oris
16 Facial vein
17 Facial artery
18 Superior labial artery
19 Orbicularis oris
20 Mentalis
21 Depressor labii inferioris
22 Depressor anguli oris
23 Platysma
24 Risorius
25 Masseter
26 Buccal branches of facial nerve
27 Buccal fat pad
28 Accessory parotid gland
29 Parotid duct
30 Transverse facial artery
31 Zygomatic branches of facial nerve
32 Zygomatic arch
33 Temporal branches of facial nerve
34 Deep part of parotid gland
35 Superficial part of parotid gland
36 Marginal mandibular branch of facial nerve
37 Cervical branch of facial nerve
38 External jugular vein
39 Great auricular nerve
40 Sternocleidomastoid
41 Lesser occipital nerve
42 Greater occipital nerve
43 Occipital artery
44 Occipital belly of occipitofrontalis
45 Occipital vein

● The parotid gland spills over from an irregular space bounded in front by the ramus of the mandible (with the attachments of masseter laterally and the medial pterygoid medially), behind by the mastoid process (with the attachments of sternocleidomastoid laterally and the posterior belly of digastric medially) and medially by the styloid process (with its three attached muscles – stylohyoid, styloglossus and stylopharyngeus). It is enclosed in a capsule derived from the investing layer of deep cervical fascia.

● Embedded within the gland are: the facial nerve, the retromandibular vein, the upper end of the external carotid artery and the beginning of its two terminal branches (the maxillary and superficial temporal arteries), lymph nodes, and filaments from the auriculotemporal nerve.

● The pathway for parotid gland secretion: from the inferior salivary nucleus by the glossopharyngeal nerve and its tympanic branch, the tympanic plexus and lesser petrosal nerve to the otic ganglion (synapse) and then to the gland by filaments of the auriculotemporal nerve.

● For the parotid gland in horizontal section see page 141.

● The main part of the epicranius muscle (a term rarely used) consists of the occipital and frontal bellies of the occipitofrontalis, united by the epicranial aponeurosis (galea aponeurotica). The temporoparietalis, which is also classified as part of the epicranius, is the name given to muscle fibres (if present) at the side of the scalp between the frontal belly of occipitofrontalis and the auricular muscles (usually small and unimportant and not illustrated here).

● The occipital belly of occipitofrontalis (see also page 99) has a bony attachment to the supreme nuchal line and the mastoid process; the frontal belly has no bony attachment.

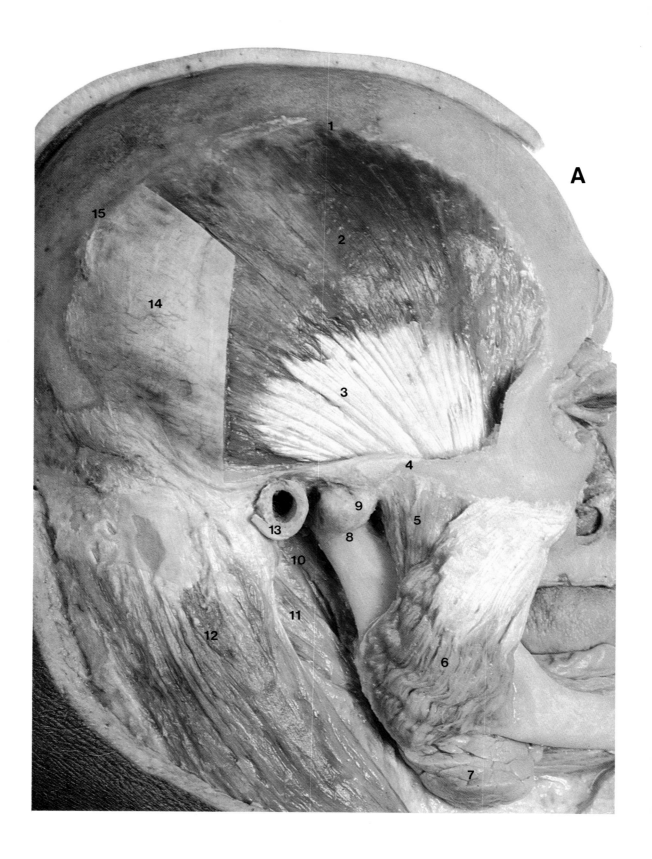

A

THE FACE

Deep dissection I

The right temporalis and masseter muscles and the temporomandibular joint

A From the right
B From the front and right, with masseter reflected

1 Inferior temporal line
2 Temporalis muscle
3 Temporalis tendon
4 Zygomatic arch
5 Middle layer   ⎫
6 Superficial layer ⎬ of masseter
7 Submandibular gland
8 Neck of mandible
9 Lateral ligament of temporomandibular joint
10 Styloid process
11 Posterior belly of digastric
12 Sternocleidomastoid
13 Cartilage of external acoustic meatus
14 Temporalis fascia
15 Superior temporal line
16 Coronoid process ⎫
17 Ramus   ⎬ of mandible
18 Medial pterygoid
19 Cut edge of mucous membrane of mouth

● The temporalis arises from the temporal fossa (except for the zygomatic arch) and from the overlying temporalis fascia (which passes from the *superior* temporal line to the zygomatic arch). The attachment of the muscle is limited above by the *inferior* temporal line.
● The insertion of temporalis is to the apex, anterior and posterior borders and medial surface of the coronoid process, and extends down the anterior border of the ramus almost as far as the third molar tooth.

● The masseter consists of three overlapping layers – superficial, arising from the zygomatic process of the maxilla and the anterior two-thirds of the lower border of the zygomatic arch; middle, arising from the deep surface of the anterior two-thirds of the arch and the lower border of the posterior third; and deep, from the deep surface of the arch. The layers fuse anteriorly and are inserted into the lateral surface of the angle, ramus and coronoid process of the mandible.

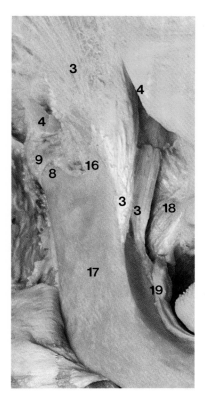

B

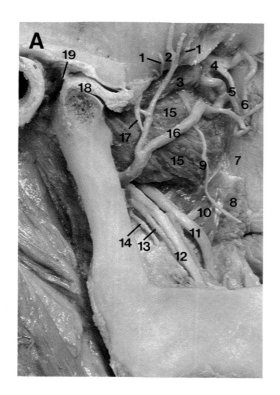

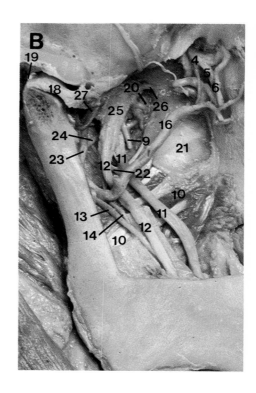

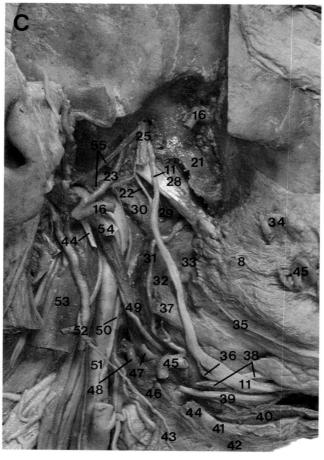

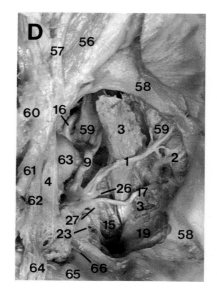

THE FACE

Deep dissection II

The right infratemporal fossa and temporomandibular joint

A **After removal of the temporalis muscle, the zygomatic arch, masseter muscle and part of the mandible**
B **After removal of the lateral pterygoid muscle**
C **After removal of the mandible, with the adjacent part of the neck**
D **From above, after removal of part of the middle cranial fossa**

 1 Deep temporal nerve
 2 Deep temporal artery
 3 Upper head of lateral pterygoid
 4 Maxillary nerve
 5 Posterior superior alveolar nerve
 6 Posterior superior alveolar artery
 7 Infratemporal surface of maxilla
 8 Buccinator
 9 Buccal nerve
10 Medial pterygoid
11 Lingual nerve
12 Inferior alveolar nerve
13 Inferior alveolar artery
14 Nerve to mylohyoid
15 Lower head of lateral pterygoid
16 Maxillary artery
17 Masseteric nerve
18 Articular disc ⎫
19 Capsule ⎬ of temporomandibular joint
21 Lateral pterygoid plate
22 Chorda tympani
23 Middle meningeal artery
24 Accessory meningeal artery
25 Mandibular nerve
26 Nerve to lateral pterygoid
27 Auriculotemporal nerve
28 Tensor veli palatini
29 Levator veli palatini
30 Pharyngobasilar fascia
31 Ascending palatine artery
32 Superior constrictor of pharynx
33 Pterygomandibular raphe
34 Parotid duct
35 Mucoperiosteum of mandible
36 Submandibular ganglion
37 Styloglossus
38 Submandibular duct
39 Hypoglossal nerve
40 Mylohyoid
41 Tendon of digastric
42 Hyoid bone
43 Thyrohyoid and nerve
44 Stylohyoid
45 Facial artery

46 Hyoglossus
47 Stylohyoid ligament
48 Lingual artery
49 Stylopharyngeus and glossopharyngeal nerve
50 Ascending pharyngeal artery
51 Internal carotid artery
52 Hypoglossal nerve hooking round occipital artery and sternocleidomastoid branch
53 Internal jugular vein
54 Styloid process
55 Roots of auriculotemporal nerve
56 Posterior part of orbit
57 Frontal nerve
58 Floor of lateral part of middle cranial fossa
59 Temporalis
60 Optic nerve
61 Oculomotor nerve
62 Ophthalmic nerve
63 Sphenoidal sinus
64 Trigeminal nerve and ganglion
65 Petrous part of temporal bone
66 Greater petrosal nerve

● The boundaries of the infratemporal fossa:
    roof – the infratemporal surface of the greater wing of the sphenoid bone containing the foramen ovale and spinosum, a small part of the squamous part of the temporal bone, and laterally the gap between the zygomatic arch and the side of the skull (forming the communication between the temporal and infratemporal fossae)
    medially – the lateral pterygoid plate
    laterally – the ramus of the mandible
    in front – the maxilla

● The contents of the infratemporal fossa:
    the temporalis and its insertion into the coronoid process of the mandible
    the medial and lateral pterygoid muscles
    the pterygoid plexus of veins
    the maxillary artery and its branches
    the mandibular nerve and its branches
    the chorda tympani

● In C the maxillary artery is seen passing through the pterygomaxillary fissure (in front of the lateral pterygoid plate) to enter the pterygopalatine fossa. For the boundaries of the fossa see page 71.

● The pterygopalatine fossa contains the maxillary artery, maxillary nerve and the pterygopalatine ganglion. For a view of the ganglion from the medial side see page 142.

● The lateral and medial pterygoid muscles both have an origin from the *lateral* pterygoid plate. (The medial pterygoid plate gives attachment to part of the superior constrictor of the pharynx.)

● The lateral pterygoid muscle helps to open the mouth by pulling the head of the mandible forwards on to the articular tubercle in front of the mandibular fossa; the other muscles of mastication (medial pterygoid, temporalis and masseter) help to close it.

● In trigeminal nerve paralysis, there is paralysis of the muscles of mastication with eventual hollowing above and below the zygomatic arch due to wasting of the temporalis and masseter.

The Orbit

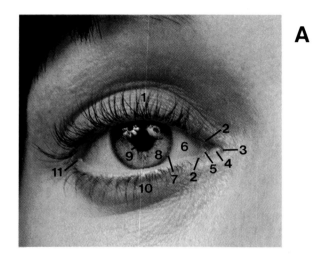

A

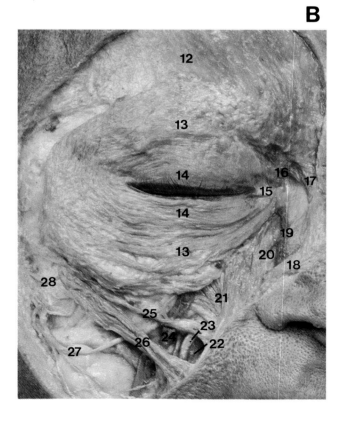

B

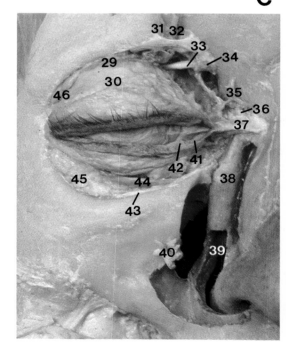

C

THE ORBIT

The eye from the front *(See also page 110)*

A The right eye

1 Upper eyelid
2 Lacrimal papilla
3 Medial angle (inner canthus)
4 Lacrimal caruncle
5 Plica semilunaris
6 Sclera with overlying conjunctiva
7 Sclerocorneal junction (limbus)
8 Iris
9 Pupil
10 Lower eyelid
11 Lateral angle (outer canthus)

B The right orbicularis oculi

12 Frontal belly of occipitofrontalis
13 Orbital part ⎫
14 Palpebral part ⎬ of orbicularis oculi
15 Medial palebral ligament
16 Depressor supercilii
17 Procerus
18 Nasalis
19 Angular vein
20 Levator labii superioris alaeque nasi
21 Levator labii superioris
22 Levator anguli oris
23 Facial artery
24 Facial vein
25 Zygomaticus minor
26 Zygomaticus major
27 Buccal ⎫
28 Zygomatic ⎬ branches of facial nerve

C Superficial dissection of the right orbit *(with removal of part of the maxilla to display the nasolacrimal duct)*

29 Muscle fibres ⎫ of levator palpebrae
30 Aponeurosis ⎬ superioris
31 Supra-orbital nerve
32 Supra-orbital artery
33 Tendon of superior oblique
34 Trochlea
35 Dorsal nasal artery
36 Lacrimal sac (upper extremity)
37 Medial palpebral ligament
38 Nasolacrimal duct
39 Opening of nasolacrimal duct (anterior wall removed)
40 Infra-orbital nerve
41 Lower lacrimal canaliculus
42 Lower lacrimal papilla and punctum
43 Cut edge of orbital septum and periosteum
44 Inferior oblique
45 Orbital fat pad
46 Lacrimal gland

● Some connective tissues of the eye and orbit:
The orbital fascia is the periosteum of the orbit (periorbita).
The orbital septum is a thin sheet of tissue continuous with the periosteum at the orbital margin, blending in the upper eyelid with the superficial lamella of the aponeurosis of levator palpebrae superioris, and in the lower eyelid with the anterior surface of the tarsus.
The lacrimal fascia stretches between the anterior and posterior lacrimal crests, covering the lacrimal sac and being pierced by the lacrimal canaliculi.
The sheath of the eyeball (fascial sheath, Tenon's capsule) envelops the eyeball from the optic nerve to the sclerocorneal junction. It is pierced by the ciliary vessels and nerves and the tendons of the eyeball muscles, being reflected on to each muscle as a sheath.
The medial and lateral check ligaments are expansions of the sheaths of the medial and lateral rectus muscles respectively that are attached to the posterior lacrimal crest (medial) and marginal tubercle (lateral).
The suspensory ligament of the eyeball is the lower part of the sheath of the eyeball, between the medial and lateral check ligaments.
The medial palpebral ligament passes from the medial ends of the two tarsi to the anterior lacrimal crest and the adjoining part of the frontal process of the maxilla. It lies in front of the lacrimal sac, with the lacrimal fascia intervening.
The lateral palpebral ligament (which is smaller than its medial fellow) passes from the lateral ends of the two tarsi to the marginal tubercle where it is attached in front of the lateral check ligament and behind the lateral palpebral raphe.
The lateral palpebral raphe is formed by interlacing fibres of the palpebral part of orbicularis oculi.

● The lacrimal apparatus consists of:
the lacrimal gland and its excretory ducts
the upper and lower lacrimal puncta opening into the lacrimal canaliculi and their dilated ampullae
the lacrimal sac receiving the canaliculi
the nasolacrimal duct, continuing downwards from the lacrimal sac and opening into the inferior meatus

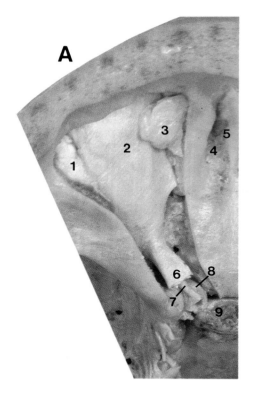

A

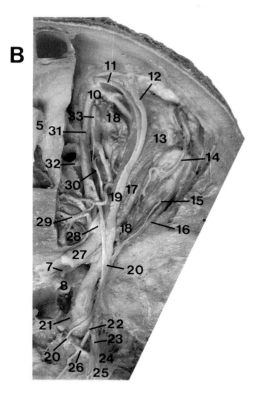

B

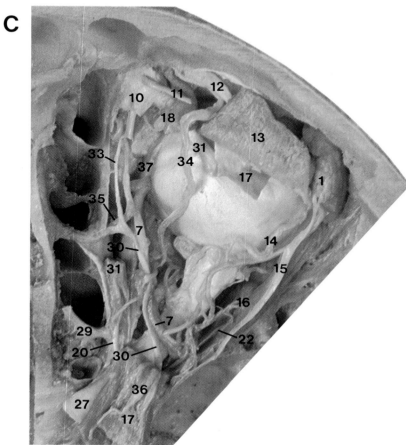

C

THE ORBIT

The orbits dissected from above

A **The left orbital periosteum**
B **Superficial dissection of the right orbit**
C **Dissection of the right orbit** *(with reflexion of levator palpebrae superioris and superior rectus) (magnified ×2)*

1 Lacrimal gland
2 Periosteum
3 Ethmoidal air cell
4 Cribriform plate of ethmoid bone
5 Crista galli
6 Dural sheath of optic nerve
7 Ophthalmic artery
8 Internal carotid artery
9 Pituitary gland
10 Trochlea
11 Supratrochlear nerve
12 Supra-orbital nerve
13 Levator palpebrae superioris
14 Lacrimal artery
15 Lacrimal nerve
16 Lateral rectus
17 Superior rectus
18 Superior ophthalmic vein
19 Frontal nerve
20 Trochlear nerve
21 Oculomotor nerve
22 Abducent nerve
23 Ophthalmic nerve
24 Trigeminal ganglion
25 Trigeminal nerve
26 Petrosphenoidal ligament
27 Optic nerve
28 Common tendinous ring
29 Posterior ethmoidal artery
30 Nasociliary nerve
31 Superior oblique
32 Anterior ethmoidal nerve
33 Infratrochlear nerve
34 Supra-orbital artery
35 Anterior ethmoidal artery
36 Superior division of oculomotor nerve
37 Medial rectus

● The supra-orbital artery, which normally arises from the ophthalmic artery near the back of the orbit, as in C, was absent in B.

● Nerve supplies of the eye and eyeball muscles:
  Motor to eyeball muscles:
    Lateral rectus by the abducent nerve
    Superior oblique by the trochlear nerve
    Other eyeball muscles (medial, superior and inferior recti and inferior oblique) by the oculomotor nerve, which also supplies levator palpebrae superioris
  Sensory:
    To the cornea: long and short ciliary nerves
    To the conjunctiva: lacrimal, supra-orbital, supratrochlear, infratrochlear and infra-orbital nerves

● Individual eyeball muscles turn the eye as follows:
  Lateral rectus: out
  Medial rectus: in
  Superior rectus: up and in
  Inferior rectus: down and in
  Superior oblique: out, and down when turned in
  Inferior oblique: out, and up when turned in
● The superior and inferior recti not only turn the eye upwards or downwards respectively but also assist the medial rectus in turning it inwards. This is because the insertions of the superior and inferior recti on the eyeball lie medial to the vertical axis.
● The superior and inferior oblique muscles not only turn the eye downwards or upwards respectively but also outwards. This is because their insertions lie lateral to the vertical axis. However, it must be noted that the depressor action of the superior oblique and the elevator action of the inferior oblique can only occur when the eye is turned in.
● Levator palpebrae superioris contains some smooth muscle fibres which receive a sympathetic nerve supply.

● Apart from the six muscles that move the eyeball (the four recti and two obliques) and the levator palpebrae superioris, there is an eighth muscle within the orbit, the orbitalis. It consists of smooth muscle that bridges over the infra-orbital groove and inferior orbital fissure, and although large in some animals it is an unimportant vestigial structure in the human orbit.

● Lesions of the motor nerves to the eyeball muscles all give varying degrees of diplopia (double vision) and strabismus (squint).
● Oculomotor nerve paralysis:
  The upper eyelid droops (ptosis), closing the eye, due to paralysis of levator palpebrae superioris (the part of the levator supplied by sympathetic fibres is not sufficient to keep the eye open).
  When the upper eyelid is lifted up, the eye is seen to be looking outwards and slightly downwards, due to the unopposed action of the lateral rectus (abducent nerve) and superior oblique (trochlear nerve).
  The eye cannot look straight upwards or downwards or inwards, due to paralysis of the superior, inferior and medial recti.
  The pupil is dilated and does not react to light or on accommodation, due to interruption of the parasympathetic fibres from the Edinger-Westphal nucleus that run in the oculomotor nerve to the ciliary ganglion and which normally act to constrict the pupil.
● Trochlear nerve paralysis:
  There is weakness when looking downwards with the eye turned in, due to paralysis of the superior oblique.
● Abducent nerve paralysis:
  The eye cannot look outwards, due to paralysis of the lateral rectus, and is deviated inwards by the unopposed action of the medial, superior and inferior recti (oculomotor nerve).

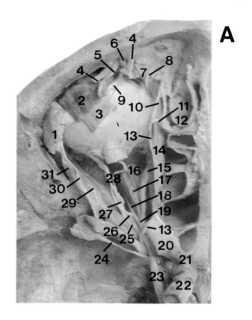

A

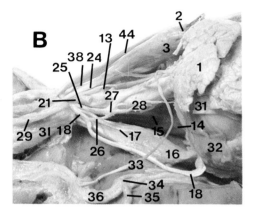

B

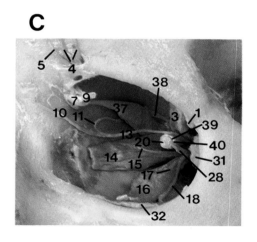

C

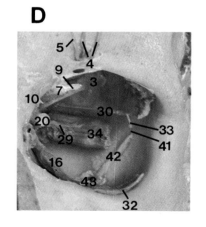

D

THE ORBIT

Deep dissection I

The ciliary ganglion and dissection from the front

A **The left orbit and ciliary ganglion, from above**
B **The right orbit and ciliary ganglion, from the
   right** (after removal of smaller blood vessels)
C **The left orbit, from the front and the left**
   (after removal of the eye)
D **The left orbit, from the front and the right**
   (after removal of the eye)

 1 Lacrimal gland
 2 Levator palpebrae superioris
 3 Superior rectus
 4 Supra-orbital nerve
 5 Supra-orbital artery
 6 Superior ophthalmic vein
 7 Trochlea
 8 Supratrochlear nerve
 9 Tendon of superior oblique
10 Infratrochlear nerve
11 Anterior ethmoidal nerve
12 Ethmoidal air cell
13 Nasociliary nerve
14 Medial rectus
15 Nerve to medial rectus
16 Inferior rectus
17 Nerve to inferior rectus
18 Nerve to inferior oblique
19 Inferior branch of oculomotor nerve
20 Optic nerve
21 Ophthalmic artery
22 Internal carotid artery
23 Oculomotor nerve
24 Superior branch of oculomotor nerve
25 Nasociliary root of ciliary ganglion
26 Oculomotor (parasympathetic) root of
   ciliary ganglion
27 Ciliary ganglion
28 Short ciliary nerves
29 Abducent nerve
30 Lacrimal nerve
31 Lateral rectus
32 Inferior oblique
33 Communication between **30** and **36** (in B)
   or **42** (in D)
34 Infra-orbital nerve
35 Infra-orbital artery
36 Maxillary nerve
37 Superior oblique
38 Trochlear nerve
39 Subarachnoid space
40 Dural sheath of optic nerve
41 Zygomatico-orbital foramen
42 Zygomatic nerve
43 Inferior orbital fissure
44 Frontal nerve

● In B the zygomatic branch of the maxillary nerve has
been removed, and the communicating branch with the
lacrimal nerve has arisen directly from the maxillary nerve.

● Ciliary arteries:
   The *anterior* ciliary arteries (variable in number) are so
      named because they arise near the front of the orbit
      from muscular branches of the ophthalmic artery, and
      run to the front of the eyeball along the tendons of the
      rectus muscles.
   The *posterior* ciliary arteries are so named because they
      arise near the back of the orbit.
   The *short posterior* ciliary arteries (about seven in
      number) run from the ophthalmic artery along the
      outside of the dural sheath of the optic nerve and
      divide into further branches before piercing the sclera
      near the nerve.
   The *long posterior* ciliary arteries (usually two) pass
      from the ophthalmic artery to pierce the sclera on
      either side of the optic nerve.

● Ciliary nerves:
   The *short* ciliary nerves (eight to ten in number) are
      branches from the ciliary ganglion that contain
      postganglionic parasympathetic fibres for the pupil
      and ciliary muscle. They also contain afferent fibres
      from the eyeball, including the cornea.
   The *long* ciliary nerves (two or three in number) are
      branches of the nasociliary nerve and contain afferent
      fibres from the eyeball, including the cornea.

● The four parasympathetic ganglia in the head and neck
are:
   the ciliary ganglion, lying in the back of the orbit on the
      lateral side of the optic nerve
   the pterygopalatine ganglion, in the pterygopalatine fossa
   the otic ganglion, on the medial side of the mandibular
      nerve just below the foramen ovale
   the submandibular ganglion, below the lingual nerve on the
      outer surface of the hyoglossus

● The direct pupillary light reflex: shining a light into one
eye causes the pupil of that eye to constrict.
   The consensual (indirect) pupillary light reflex: shining a
light into one eye causes the pupil of the *opposite* eye to
constrict.
   The pathway for the pupillary light reflexes: from the retina
by the optic nerve, chiasma and tract to the pretectal nucleus
(synapse) at the level of the superior colliculus, then to the
Edinger-Westphal part of the oculomotor nucleus and by the
inferior division of the oculomotor nerve and the branch to the
inferior oblique to reach the ciliary ganglion (synapse), and
then by short ciliary nerves to the sphincter pupillae. The
pupils of both eyes constrict because (a) some fibres cross in
the optic chiasma, and (b) fibres from the pretectal nucleus
pass to the Edinger-Westphal nuclei of both sides.

● Possible pathways for the accommodation-convergence
reflexes (for looking at near objects):
   For accommodation: from the visual cortex by the posterior
limb of the internal capsule to the Edinger-Westphal nucleus
(*not* via the pretectal nucleus) and so to the ciliary ganglion,
sphincter pupillae and ciliary muscle as for the pupillary light
reflexes.
   For convergence: from the visual cortex by association
fibres to the frontal eye field (middle frontal gyrus) (synapse),
then by the anterior limb of the internal capsule to those cells
of the oculomotor nucleus that supply the medial rectus.

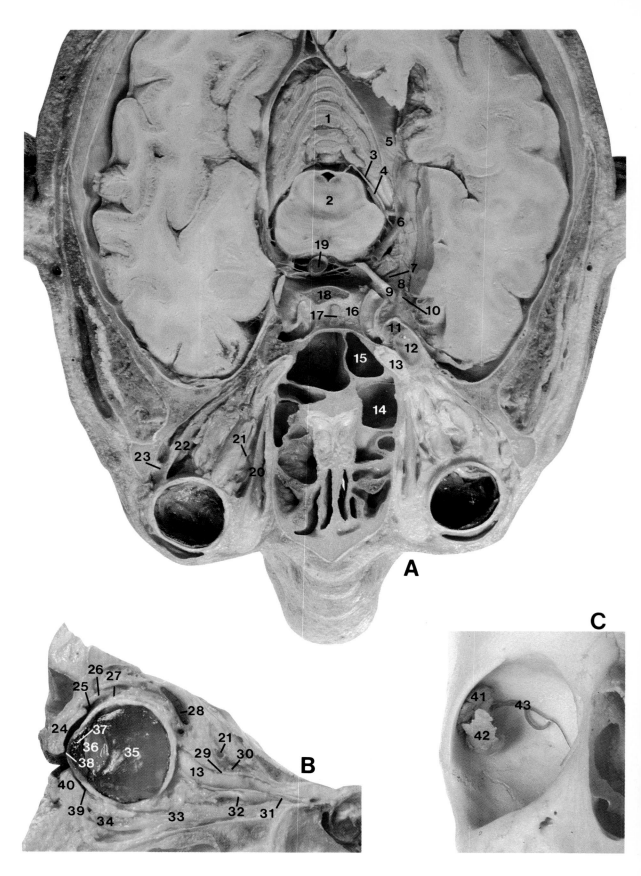

THE ORBIT

Deep dissection II

Transverse and sagittal sections, the lacrimal gland and the eye

A Transverse section through the orbits and the nasal and cranial cavities, from above
B Sagittal section through the right orbit, from the left

1 Cerebellum
2 Junction of pons and midbrain
3 Trochlear nerve
4 Superior cerebellar artery
5 Tentorium cerebelli
6 Posterior cerebral artery
7 Attached margin of tentorium cerebelli
8 Roof of cavernous sinus
9 Oculomotor nerve
10 Free margin of tentorium cerebelli
11 Anterior clinoid process
12 Extension of posterior ethmoidal air cell into lesser wing of sphenoid bone
13 Optic nerve
14 Posterior ethmoidal air cell
15 Sphenoidal sinus
16 Diaphragma sellae
17 Pituitary stalk
18 Dorsum sellae
19 Basilar artery
20 Medial rectus
21 Ophthalmic artery
22 Lateral rectus
23 Lateral check ligament
24 Superior tarsus
25 Superior conjunctival fornix
26 Levator palpebrae superioris
27 Tendon of superior rectus
28 Superior ophthalmic vein
29 Dural sheath of optic nerve
30 Nasociliary nerve
31 Central artery of retina
32 Inferior ophthalmic vein
33 Inferior rectus
34 Inferior oblique
35 Vitreous humour
36 Lens
37 Anterior chamber
38 Cornea
39 Inferior conjunctival fornix
40 Inferior tarsus

● The lacrimal gland has an upper (larger) orbital part and a lower (smaller) palpebral part, continuous with each other round the lateral (concave) border of the aponeurosis of levator palpebrae superioris.
● The orbital part lies in the lacrimal fossa of the frontal bone, above the levator.
● The palpebral part lies below the levator and extends into the lateral part of the upper eyelid.
● About 12 small ducts open into the superior conjunctival fornix, those from the orbital part passing through the palpebral part.
● The pathway for lacrimal gland secretion: from the superior salivary nucleus by the nervus intermedius part of the facial nerve, greater petrosal nerve and nerve of the pterygoid canal to the pterygopalatine ganglion (synapse) and then to the gland by the maxillary nerve, its zygomatic branch and the communication with the lacrimal nerve.

The lacrimal gland

C An isolated right lacrimal gland, replaced within the orbit, from the left and below

41 Orbital part
42 Palpebral part
43 Lacrimal artery and nerve

The lens and ciliary body of the eye, from behind *(in the anterior half of an eyeball sectioned through the equator) (magnified ×1.5)*

D With the lens in situ
E With the lens removed

44 Retina (optic part)
45 Choroid
46 Sclera
47 Ora serrata
48 Ciliary part of retina
49 Posterior surface of lens
50 Ciliary processes
51 Margin of pupil
52 Posterior surface of cornea

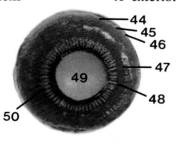

D

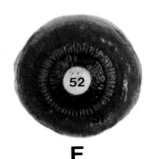

E

The Nose

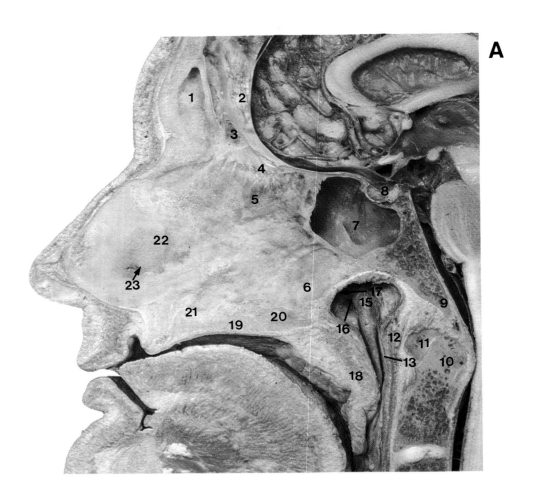

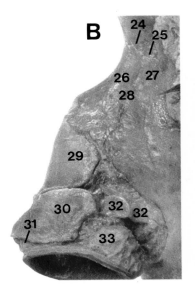

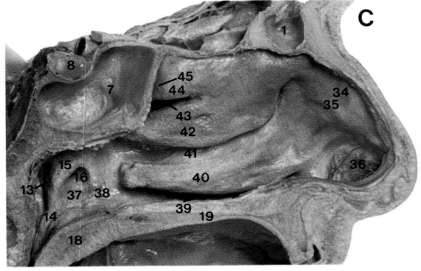

THE NOSE

The nasal cartilages and the nasal cavity *(For surface markings of the external nose see page 110)*

A The nasal septum, from the left
B The skeleton of the external nose, from the left
C The lateral wall of the left nasal cavity and nasopharynx
D As C, with a supreme nasal concha

1 Frontal sinus
2 Falx cerebri
3 Crista galli
4 Cribriform plate of ethmoid bone and filaments of olfactory nerve
5 Perpendicular plate of ethmoid bone
6 Vomer
7 Sphenoidal sinus
8 Pituitary gland
9 Anterior margin of foramen magnum
10 Dens of axis
11 Anterior arch of atlas
12 Pharyngeal tonsil
13 Pharyngeal recess
14 Salpingopharyngeal fold
15 Tubal elevation
16 Opening of auditory tube
17 Right choana (posterior nasal aperture)
18 Soft palate
19 Hard palate
20 Nasal crest of palatine bone
21 Nasal crest of maxilla
22 Septal cartilage
23 Vomeronasal organ
24 Frontonasal suture
25 Frontomaxillary suture
26 Nasal bone
27 Frontal process of maxilla
28 Nasomaxillary suture
29 Lateral nasal cartilage
30 Greater nasal cartilage
31 Septal process (medial crus) of greater nasal cartilage
32 Lesser alar cartilages
33 Fibrofatty tissue
34 Atrium
35 Agger nasi
36 Vestibule
37 Levator elevation
38 Salpingopalatal fold
39 Inferior meatus
40 Inferior nasal concha
41 Middle meatus
42 Middle nasal concha
43 Superior meatus
44 Superior nasal concha
45 Spheno-ethmoidal recess
46 Supreme nasal concha
47 Supreme meatus

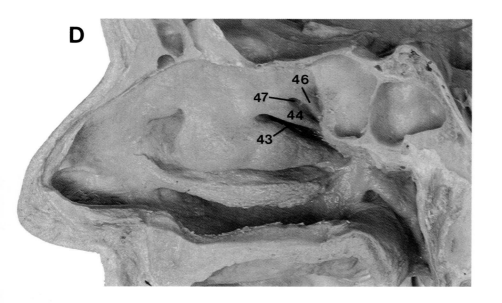

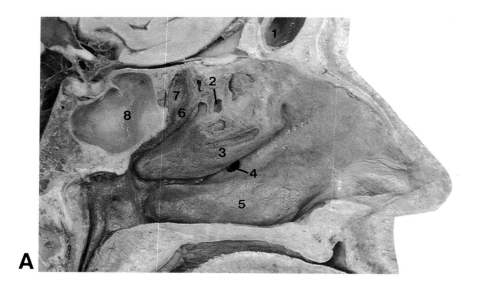

A

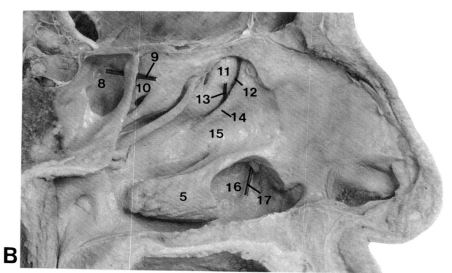

B

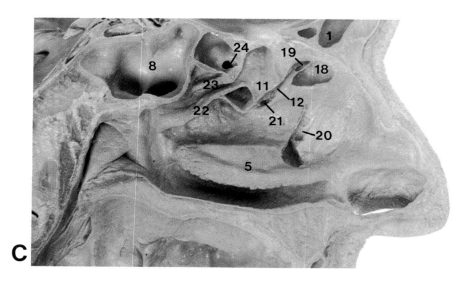

C

128

THE NOSE

The lateral wall of the left nasal cavity

A **The lateral wall of the left half of the nasal cavity** *(with removal of the superior and part of the middle nasal conchae)*
B **With removal of the middle and part of the inferior nasal conchae**
C **With removal of parts of the nasal conchae and opening up of the lower end of the nasolacrimal duct**

1 Frontal sinus
2 A middle ethmoidal air cell
3 Middle nasal concha
4 Unusually low aperture of maxillary sinus
5 Inferior nasal concha
6 Superior nasal concha
7 Spheno-ethmoidal recess
8 Sphenoidal sinus
9 Bristle in aperture of sphenoidal sinus
10 Supreme nasal concha
11 Ethmoidal bulla
12 Semilunar hiatus
13 Bristle in aperture of maxillary sinus
14 Mucous membrane overlying uncinate process of ethmoid bone
15 Middle meatus
16 Inferior meatus
17 Bristle in opening of nasolacrimal duct
18 An anterior ethmoidal air cell
19 Frontonasal duct
20 Lower end of nasolacrimal duct
21 Aperture of maxillary sinus
22 Base of middle nasal concha
23 Base of superior nasal concha
24 Aperture of a posterior ethmoidal air cell

D **Nerves of the lateral wall of the right half of the nasal cavity** *(with removal of the posterior parts of the nasal conchae and part of the perpendicular plate of the palatine bone to display the greater palatine canal)* *(For nerves of the nasal septum see page 135)*

25 Olfactory nerve filaments
26 Sphenopalatine artery and foramen
27 Pterygopalatine ganglion
28 A lateral posterior superior nasal nerve
29 Greater palatine nerve and canal
30 A posterior inferior nasal nerve
31 Vestibule of nose
32 Anterior ethmoidal nerve

● The frontal sinus opens into the middle meatus by the frontonasal duct.
● The anterior ethmoidal air cells open into the frontonasal duct or the infundibulum (the upward anterior continuation of the semilunar hiatus) in the middle meatus.
● The middle ethmoidal air cells open on or above the ethmoidal bulla in the middle meatus.
● The posterior ethmoidal air cells open into the superior meatus.
● The sphenoidal sinus opens into the spheno-ethmoidal recess.
● The maxillary sinus opens into the semilunar hiatus in the middle meatus.
● The nasolacrimal duct opens into the inferior meatus.

● Opening into the superior meatus: posterior ethmoidal air cells.
● Opening into the middle meatus: the frontal sinus, anterior and middle ethmoidal air cells and the maxillary sinus.
● Opening into the inferior meatus: the nasolacrimal duct.
● Opening into the spheno-ethmoidal recess: the sphenoidal sinus.

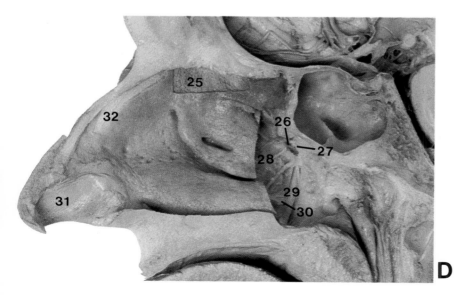

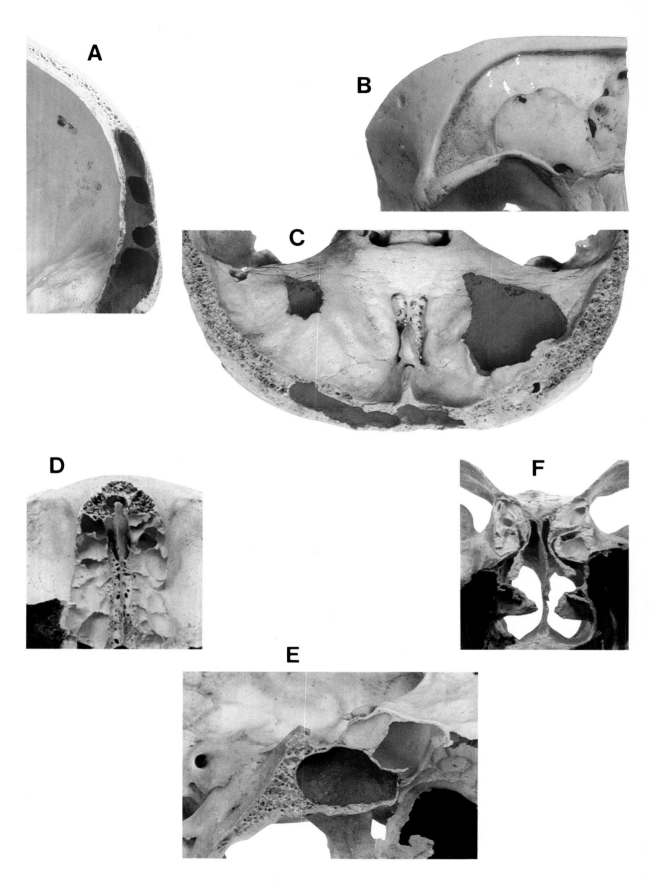

THE NOSE

The paranasal sinuses, in sections of parts of the skull *(Frontal sinus, red; ethmoidal sinus, yellow; sphenoidal sinus, dark blue; maxillary sinus, green; middle nasal concha, brown; inferior nasal concha, light blue)*

The frontal sinuses

A **A sagittal section of a large left sinus** *(extending high in the squamous part of the frontal bone)*
B **A right sinus dissected out of the diploë, from the front**
C **Two large sinuses opened from above** *(extending far back in the orbital part of the frontal bone)*

The ethmoidal sinuses

D **The roof of the ethmoidal sinuses** *(showing in the left sinus some anterior ethmoidal air cells lying in front of the lowest part of the frontal sinus)*
E **A sagittal section of unusually large left posterior ethmoidal air cells** *(overlapping the left sphenoidal sinus)*
F **The ethmoidal sinuses in coronal section** *(showing the ethmoidal bulla overlapped by the middle nasal concha)*

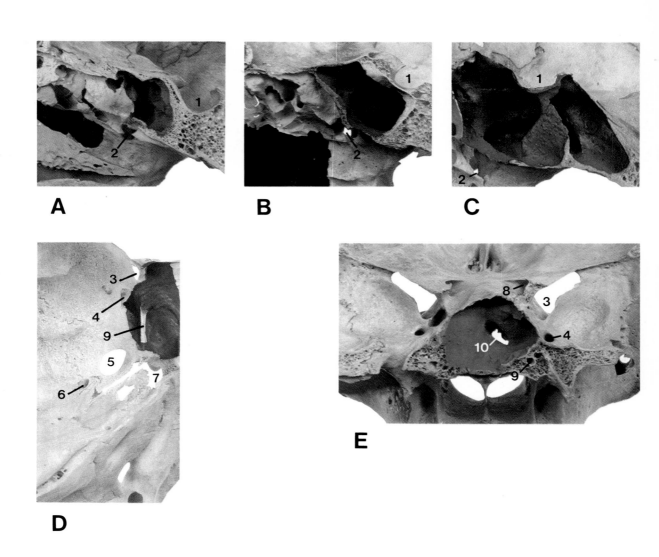

A

B

C

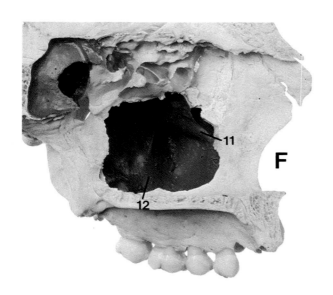

D

E

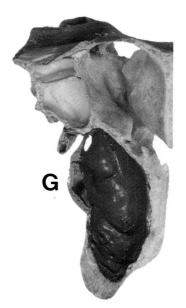

F

G

THE NOSE

The paranasal sinuses, in sections of parts of the skull *(Ethmoidal sinus, yellow; sphenoidal sinus, dark blue; maxillary sinus, green; middle nasal concha, brown; inferior nasal concha, light blue)*

The sphenoidal sinuses

A A small right sinus *(lying in front of the pituitary fossa)*

B A medium-sized sinus *(lying in front of and below the pituitary fossa)*

C A large sinus *(extending behind the pituitary fossa and into the basilar part of the occipital bone)*

D The floor of the left sinus, from above and behind *(with part of the pterygoid canal opened up (white))*

E A coronal section, from behind *(showing a very large right sinus with its aperture opening anteriorly, and a very small left sinus)*

The maxillary sinuses

F A left sinus, with the medial wall of the maxilla removed *(showing the elevation produced by the roots of the second molar tooth and the projection caused by the infra-orbital canal)*

G A right sinus in a coronal section, from the front *(showing the aperture high up in the medial wall, opening under cover of the middle nasal concha)*

H A coronal section through a small right sinus, from the front *(without any extension into the alveolar process)*

J A left sinus in a coronal section, from behind *(showing the projection of the infra-orbital canal into the roof of the sinus and the extension of the sinus into the alveolar process of the maxilla)*

1 Pituitary fossa	**7** Foramen lacerum
2 Sphenopalatine foramen	**8** Optic canal
3 Superior orbital fissure	**9** Pterygoid canal
4 Foramen rotundum	**10** Aperture of sphenoidal sinus
5 Foramen ovale	**11** Projection of infra-orbital canal
6 Foramen spinosum	**12** Elevation over molar tooth

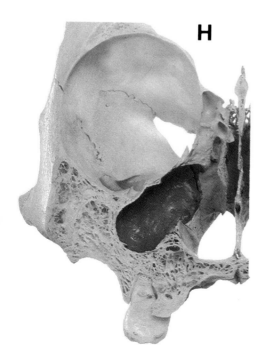

H

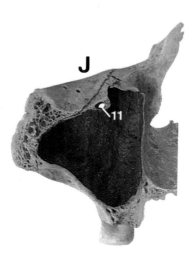

J

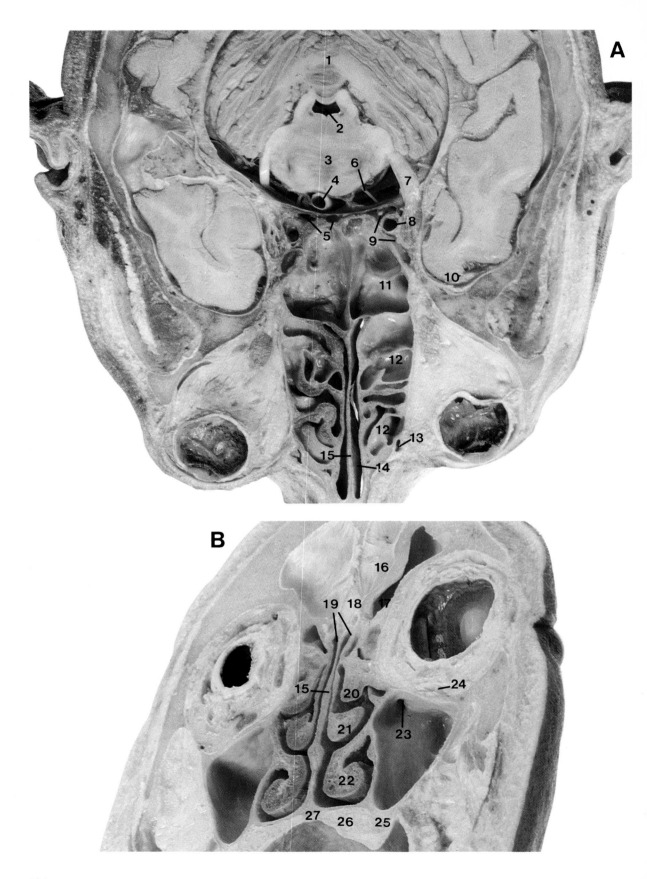

THE NOSE

Transverse and coronal sections, and nerves of the nasal septum

A Transverse section of the head at the level of the palpebral fissure, from above
B Coronal section of the head through the eyeballs, from the right, behind and below

1 Cerebellum
2 Upper part of fourth ventricle
3 Pons
4 Basilar artery
5 Basilar sinus
6 Abducent nerve
7 Trigeminal nerve
8 Internal carotid artery
9 Cavernous sinus
10 Temporal pole
11 Sphenoidal sinus
12 Ethmoidal air cells
13 Nasolacrimal duct
14 Nasal cavity
15 Nasal septum
16 Dura mater of anterior wall of anterior cranial fossa
17 Frontal sinus
18 Crista galli
19 Roof of nasal cavity
20 Superior ⎫
21 Middle ⎬ nasal concha
22 Inferior ⎭
23 Aperture of maxillary sinus
24 Infra-orbital nerve
25 Alveolar process ⎫
26 Palatine process ⎬ of maxilla
27 Hard palate

C Nerves of the left side of the nasal septum
(For nerves of the lateral wall of the nasal cavity see page 129)

28 Olfactory nerve filaments
29 Nasopalatine nerve
30 Incisive canal
31 Anterior ethmoidal nerve

● Nerves of the lateral wall of the nose:
   Olfactory (over the superior nasal concha)
   Infra-orbital (to the skin of the vestibule)
   Anterior ethmoidal
   Nasal branch of anterior superior alveolar (to part of the inferior meatus)
   Lateral posterior superior nasal
   Posterior inferior nasal

● Nerves of the nasal septum:
   Olfactory (over an area opposite the superior nasal concha)
   Anterior ethmoidal
   Medial posterior superior nasal
   Nasopalatine

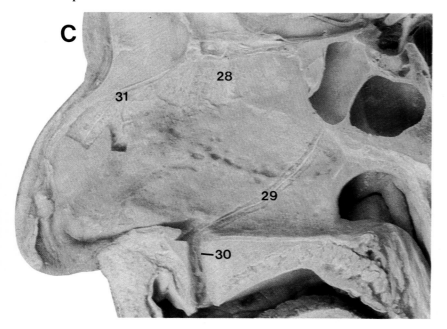

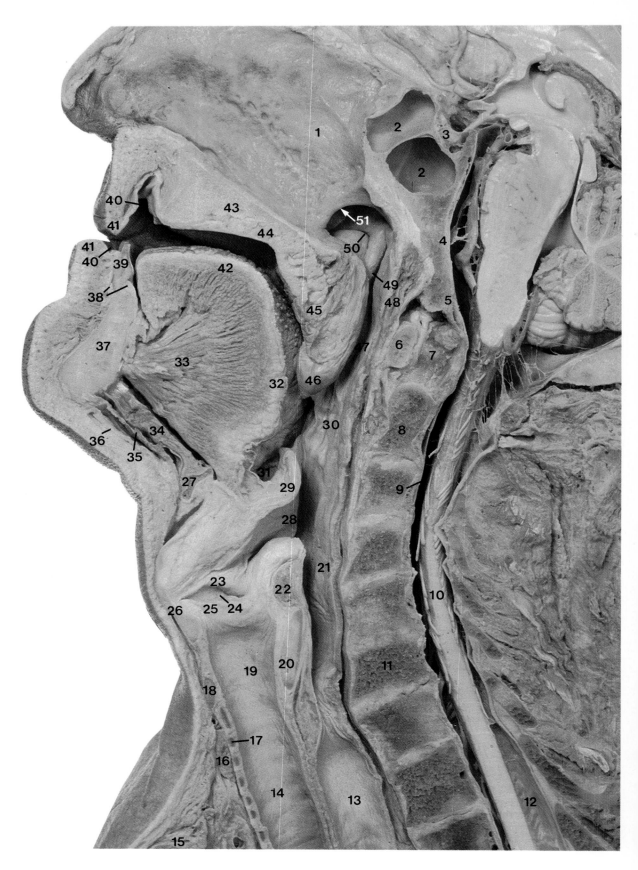

The Mouth, Palate and Pharynx

The mouth, palate, pharynx and larynx

The right half of a sagittal section of the lower part of the head and neck, slightly to the left of the midline *(For further details of the head in this specimen see page 158)*

1 Nasal septum
2 Sphenoidal sinus
3 Pituitary gland
4 Clivus
5 Anterior margin of foramen magnum
6 Anterior arch of atlas
7 Dens of axis
8 Body of axis
9 Spinal subarachnoid space
10 Spinal cord
11 Body of sixth cervical vertebra
12 Subarachnoid septum
13 Oesophagus
14 Trachea
15 Jugular notch of manubrium of sternum
16 Isthmus of thyroid gland
17 Second tracheal ring
18 Arch of cricoid cartilage
19 Lower part of larynx
20 Lamina of cricoid cartilage
21 Laryngeal part of pharynx
22 Transverse arytenoid muscle
23 Vestibular fold
24 Ventricle of larynx
25 Vocal fold (vocal cord)
26 Lamina of thyroid cartilage
27 Body of hyoid bone
28 Aryepiglottic fold
29 Epiglottis and epiglottic cartilage
30 Oral part of pharynx
31 Vallecula
32 Postsulcal part of dorsum of tongue
33 Genioglossus
34 Geniohyoid
35 Mylohyoid
36 Platysma
37 Body of mandible
38 Gingiva
39 Left lower central incisor tooth
40 Vestibule of mouth
41 Lip
42 Presulcal part of dorsum of tongue
43 Hard palate
44 Palatal glands in mucoperiosteum
45 Soft palate
46 Uvula
47 Nasal part of pharynx
48 Pharyngeal tonsil
49 Pharyngeal recess
50 Opening of auditory tube
51 Posterior nasal aperture (choana)

● The hyoid bone lies at the level of the third cervical vertebra.
● The thyroid cartilage lies at the level of the fourth and fifth cervical vertebrae.
● The cricoid cartilage lies at the level of the sixth cervical vertebra.
● The isthmus of the thyroid gland lies opposite the second, third and fourth tracheal rings.

● When enlarged the lymphoid tissue of the pharyngeal tonsil becomes known as the adenoids.

● The mouth or oral cavity consists of the vestibule and the oral cavity proper.
● The vestibule of the mouth is the narrow space bounded on the outer side by the lips and cheeks, and inside by the gingivae (gums) and teeth.
● The oral cavity proper is bounded at each side and in front by the alveolar arches with the teeth and gingivae; at the back it communicates with the oral part of the pharynx by the oropharyngeal isthmus which lies between the palatoglossal arches. (The tonsils which lie behind the palatoglossal arches are therefore in the oral part of the pharynx, not in the mouth).

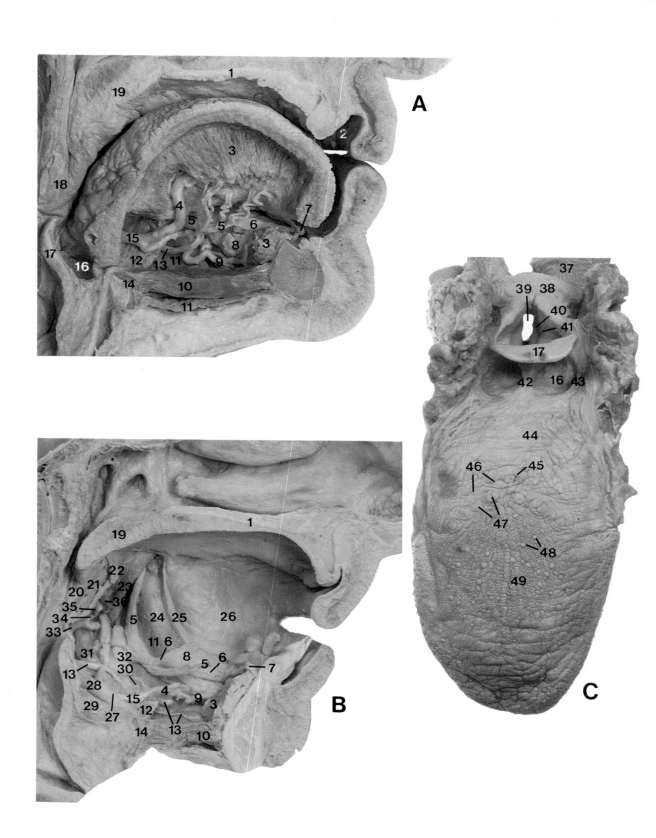

THE MOUTH, PALATE AND PHARYNX

The tongue and the floor of the mouth

A **Deep dissection of the left half of the tongue, from the right**
B **The left half of the mouth, from the right, with the tongue removed**
C **The tongue from above, with the inlet (aditus) of the larynx**

1 Hard palate
2 Vestibule of mouth
3 Genioglossus
4 Deep lingual artery
5 Lingual nerve
6 Submandibular duct
7 Orifice of submandibular duct on sublingual papilla
8 Sublingual gland
9 Sublingual artery
10 Geniohyoid
11 Mylohyoid
12 Hyoglossus
13 Hypoglossal nerve
14 Body of hyoid bone
15 Lingual artery
16 Vallecula
17 Epiglottis
18 Oral part of pharynx
19 Soft palate
20 Palatopharyngeal arch
21 Tonsil
22 Upper end of palatoglossal arch
23 Medial pterygoid
24 Upper border of body of edentulous mandible
25 Cut edge of mucous membrane
26 Mucous membrane overlying buccinator
27 Lower end of stylohyoid ligament
28 Middle constrictor of pharynx
29 Greater horn of hyoid bone
30 Vena comitans of hypoglossal nerve
31 Stylohyoid
32 Deep part of submandibular gland
33 Facial artery
34 Ascending palatine artery
35 External palatine (paratonsillar) vein
36 Styloglossus
37 Posterior wall of pharynx
38 Posterior wall of larynx
39 Rima of glottis
40 Vocal fold
41 Vestibular fold
42 Median glosso-epiglottic fold
43 Lateral glosso-epiglottic fold
44 Postsulcal part of dorsum of tongue
45 Foramen caecum
46 Sulcus terminalis
47 Vallate papillae
48 Fungiform papillae
49 Presulcal part of dorsum of tongue

● All the muscles of the tongue are supplied by the hypoglossal nerve except palatoglossus which is supplied by the pharyngeal plexus.
● The mucous membrane of the anterior two-thirds of the tongue is supplied by the lingual nerve (ordinary sensation) with chorda tympani fibres (which joined the lingual nerve in the infratemporal fossa) supplying taste buds.
● The mucous membrane of the posterior one-third of the tongue (but including the vallate papillae which lie in front of the sulcus terminalis) is supplied by the glossopharyngeal nerve (ordinary sensation *and* taste).
● The mucous membrane of the part of the tongue that lies in front of the vallecula is supplied (like the vallecula) by the internal laryngeal nerve.
● The cell bodies of the taste fibres in the chorda tympani are in the genicular ganglion of the facial nerve; of those in the glossopharyngeal nerve, in the glossopharyngeal ganglia; and of those in the internal laryngeal nerve, in the inferior vagal ganglion. The central fibres from these ganglia all converge to synapse with the cells of the nucleus of the tractus solitarius.

● The sublingual gland lies beneath the mucous membrane of the floor of the mouth, contacting the sublingual fossa of the mandible (above the mylohyoid line).
● Important relations include:
above – the mucous membrane of the floor of the mouth
below – the mylohyoid
in front – the sublingual gland of the opposite side
behind – the deep part of the submandibular gland
laterally – the sublingual fossa of the mandible (above the mylohyoid line)
medially – the genioglossus, with the lingual nerve and the submandibular duct intervening
● Small sublingual ducts (up to 20 in number) open separately in the floor of the mouth on the summit of the sublingual fold, but some of them may open instead into the submandibular duct.

● The pathway for submandibular and sublingual gland secretion: from the superior salivary nucleus by the nervus intermedius part of the facial nerve, chorda tympani and lingual nerve to the submandibular ganglion (synapse) and then to the glands by lingual nerve filaments.

● For notes on the parotid gland see page 113, and on the submandibular gland see page 141.

● The foramen caecum marks the position of the upper end of the thyroglossal duct and thyroid diverticulum, the embryonic downgrowth from which the thyroid gland develops.
● The pyramidal lobe of the thyroid gland represents a differentiation of part of the remains of the duct; other parts of the duct may persist to form cysts or aberrant masses of thyroid tissue, e.g. a lingual thyroid in the tongue.

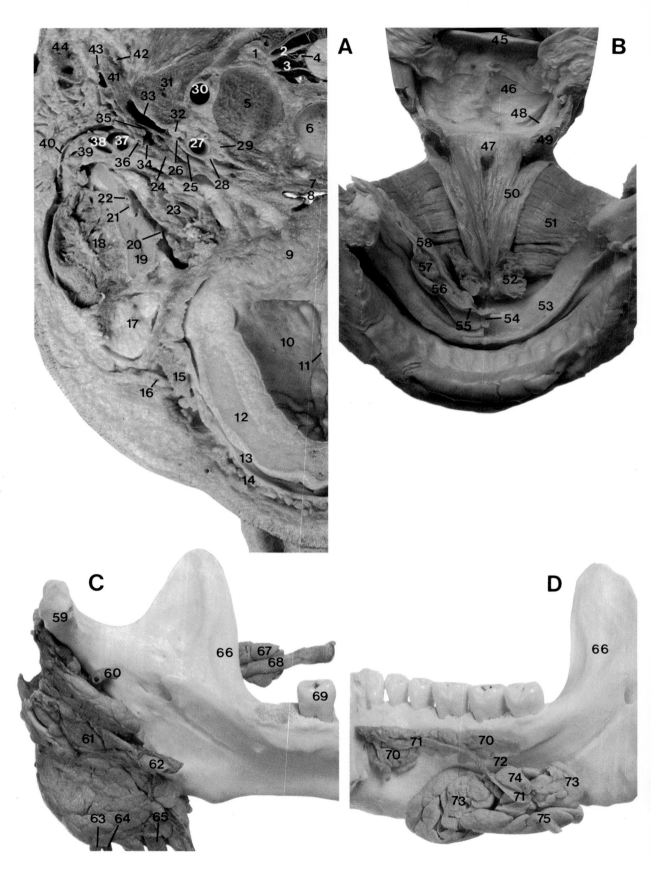

THE MOUTH, PALATE AND PHARYNX

The roof and floor of the mouth and the salivary glands

A   The left half of the roof of the mouth, mandible and parotid gland in a horizontal section of the head

1 Dorsal root ganglion ⎫
2 Dorsal root   ⎬ of second
3 Ventral root   ⎭ cervical nerve
4 Spinal root of accessory nerve
5 Lateral mass of atlas
6 Dens of axis
7 Superior constrictor of pharynx
8 Nasal part of pharynx
9 Soft palate
10 Hard palate
11 Palatal raphe
12 Alveolar process of maxilla
13 Vestibule of mouth
14 Labial glands
15 Buccinator
16 Facial artery
17 Buccal fat pad
18 Masseter
19 Ramus of mandible
20 Lingual nerve
21 Inferior alveolar nerve
22 Inferior alveolar artery
23 Medial pterygoid
24 Styloglossus
25 Stylopharyngeus
26 Glossopharyngeal nerve
27 Internal carotid artery
28 Hypoglossal nerve
29 Superior cervical sympathetic ganglion
30 Vertebral artery
31 Transverse process of atlas
32 Vagus nerve
33 Internal jugular vein
34 Stylohyoid ligament
35 Stylohyoid
36 Posterior auricular artery
37 External carotid artery
38 Retromandibular vein
39 Parotid gland
40 A zygomatic branch of facial nerve
41 Posterior belly of digastric
42 Accessory nerve
43 Occipital artery
44 Sternocleidomastoid

B   The floor of the mouth (*with the tongue removed, together with the gingiva on the left*)

45 Epiglottis
46 Vallecula
47 Body   ⎫
48 Greater horn   ⎬ of hyoid bone
49 Hyoglossus
50 Geniohyoid
51 Mylohyoid
52 Genioglossus
53 Edentulous body of mandible
54 Frenulum of tongue
55 Sublingual papilla
56 Sublingual fold
57 Sublingual gland
58 Submandibular duct

C   Isolated left parotid gland and the mandible, from the medial side (*For the lateral surface of the gland see page 112*)

D   Isolated right sublingual and submandibular glands and the mandible, from the medial side

59 Condylar process of mandible
60 Maxillary artery
61 Parotid gland
62 External carotid artery
63 Great auricular nerve
64 Posterior division ⎫
65 Anterior division ⎬ of retromandibular vein
66 Ramus of mandible
67 Accessory parotid gland
68 Parotid duct
69 Lower second molar tooth
70 Sublingual gland
71 Submandibular duct
72 Mylohyoid line of body of mandible
73 Main part ⎫
74 Deep part ⎬ of submandibular gland
75 Facial artery

● The submandibular gland has a large superficial and small deep part, continuous round the posterior border of mylohyoid.
● The superficial part lies in the digastric triangle. Important relations include:
  below – skin, platysma, the investing layer of deep cervical fascia, the facial vein, the cervical branch of the facial nerve, submandibular lymph nodes.
  laterally – the submandibular fossa of the mandible (below the mylohyoid line), the insertion of the medial pterygoid, the facial artery.
  medially – the mylohyoid and vessels, the lingual nerve and submandibular ganglion, the hypoglossal nerve, the deep lingual vein, the hyoglossus.
● The deep part of the gland lies on hyoglossus with the lingual nerve above, and the hypoglossal nerve and the submandibular duct below.

● The submandibular duct is 5cm long. It emerges from the superficial part of the gland near the posterior border of mylohyoid and passes forward between mylohyoid and hyoglossus and then between the sublingual gland and genioglossus. It opens in the floor of the mouth on the sublingual papilla at the side of the frenulum of the tongue.

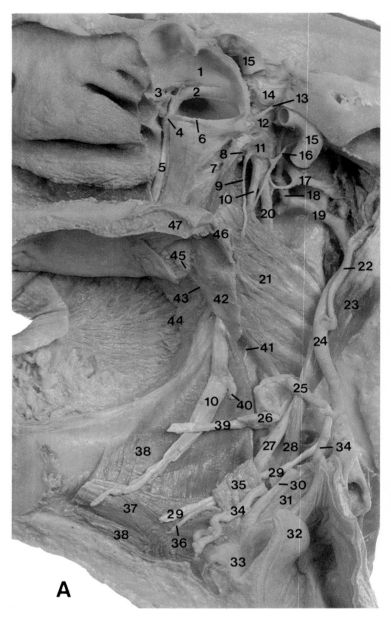

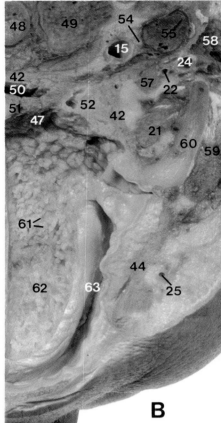

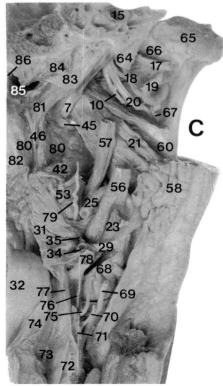

THE MOUTH, PALATE AND PHARYNX

The inside of the mouth and the hard and soft palates

A The right half of the mouth, from the left *(with skull dissection to show the trigeminal, pterygopalatine and otic ganglia)*
B The left half of the roof of the mouth, from below *(in a horizontal section through the head below the level of the hard palate)*
C The right half of the soft palate, from behind *(in a deep dissection with adjacent structures after removal of much of the pharynx)*

1 Sphenoidal sinus
2 Maxillary nerve
3 Sphenopalatine foramen and artery
4 Pterygopalatine ganglion
5 Greater palatine nerve
6 Nerve of pterygoid canal
7 Tensor veli palatini
8 Nerve to tensor veli palatini
9 Nerve to medial pterygoid
10 Lingual nerve
11 Otic ganglion
12 Mandibular nerve
13 Greater petrosal nerve
14 Trigeminal ganglion
15 Internal carotid artery
16 Chorda tympani
17 Auriculotemporal nerve
18 Middle meningeal artery
19 Maxillary artery
20 Inferior alveolar nerve
21 Medial pterygoid
22 Occipital artery
23 Posterior belly of digastric
24 External carotid artery
25 Facial artery
26 Deep part of submandibular gland
27 Tendon of digastric
28 Stylohyoid
29 Hypoglossal nerve
30 Stylohyoid ligament
31 Middle constrictor of pharynx
32 Epiglottis
33 Vallecula
34 Lingual artery
35 Hyoglossus
36 Vena comitans of hypoglossal nerve
37 Geniohyoid
38 Mylohyoid
39 Submandibular duct
40 Submandibular ganglion
41 Nerve to mylohyoid
42 Superior constrictor of pharynx
43 Pterygomandibular raphe
44 Buccinator
45 Pterygoid hamulus
46 Palatopharyngeus

47 Soft palate
48 Dens of axis
49 Lateral mass of atlas
50 Nasal part of pharynx
51 Uvula
52 Tonsil
53 Stylopharyngeus
54 Vagus nerve
55 Internal jugular vein
56 Stylohyoid
57 Styloglossus
58 Parotid gland
59 Masseter
60 Ramus of mandible
61 Palatal glands
62 Hard palate
63 Vestibule of mouth
64 Base of styloid process
65 Intra-articular disc of temporomandibular joint
66 Lateral pterygoid
67 Inferior alveolar artery
68 Posterior part of submandibular gland
69 Superior thyroid artery
70 Superior laryngeal artery
71 Inferior constrictor of pharynx
72 Lamina of thyroid cartilage
73 Piriform fossa
74 Aryepiglottic fold
75 Internal laryngeal nerve
76 Thyrohyoid
77 Thyrohyoid membrane
78 Greater horn of hyoid bone
79 Glossopharyngeal nerve
80 Palatine aponeurosis
81 Levator veli palatini
82 Musculus uvulae
83 Cartilaginous part of auditory tube
84 Longus capitis
85 Posterior nasal aperture (choana)
86 Nasal septum (vomer)

● All the muscles of the palate are supplied by the pharyngeal plexus except tensor veli palatini which is supplied by the nerve to the medial pterygoid (mandibular nerve).
● The mucous membrane of the palate is supplied by the nasopalatine, greater and lesser palatine and glossopharyngeal nerves.

● The surface of the tonsil is pitted by downgrowths of the epithelium to form the tonsillar crypts.
● A deep crypt-like structure near the upper pole of the tonsil is the intratonsillar cleft, and represents the proximal end of the embryonic second pharyngeal pouch.
● The mucous membrane on the surface of the tonsil is supplied by the glossopharyngeal and lesser palatine nerves.

● After entering the oral cavity beneath the lower border of the superior constrictor of the pharynx, the lingual nerve lies in contact with the periosteum of the mandible immediately below and behind the third molar tooth.

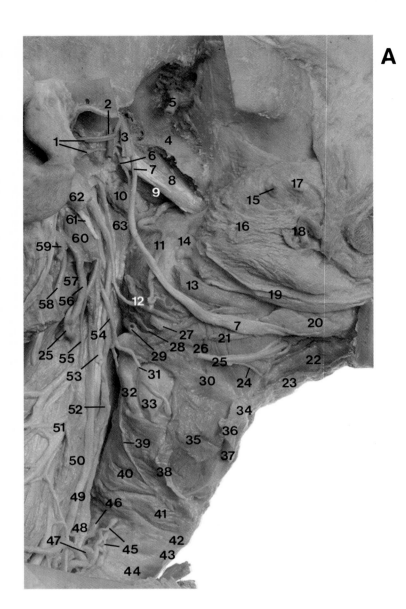

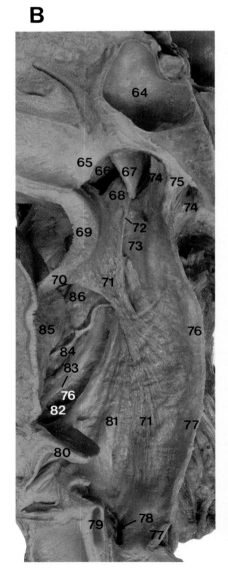

THE MOUTH, PALATE AND PHARYNX

The pharynx – external and internal surfaces

A **The external surface, from the right** (*after deep dissection of the right infratemporal fossa and neck*)

1 Roots of auriculotemporal nerve
2 Middle meningeal artery
3 Mandibular nerve
4 Lateral pterygoid plate
5 Maxillary artery entering pterygomaxillary fissure
6 Chorda tympani
7 Lingual nerve
8 Tensor veli palatini
9 Levator veli palatini
10 Pharyngobasilar fascia
11 Superior constrictor of pharynx and ascending palatine artery
12 Stylopharyngeus and glossopharyngeal nerve
13 Styloglossus
14 Pterygomandibular raphe
15 Parotid duct
16 Buccinator
17 Molar glands
18 Facial artery
19 Mucoperiosteum of mandible
20 Sublingual gland
21 Submandibular duct
22 Geniohyoid
23 Mylohyoid
24 Nerve to geniohyoid
25 Hypoglossal nerve
26 Hyoglossus
27 Stylohyoid ligament
28 Middle constrictor of pharynx
29 Lingual artery
30 Greater horn of hyoid bone
31 Internal laryngeal nerve
32 Superior horn of thyroid cartilage
33 Thyrohyoid membrane
34 Body of hyoid bone
35 Thyrohyoid
36 Superior belly of omohyoid
37 Sternohyoid
38 Sternothyroid
39 External laryngeal nerve
40 Inferior constrictor of pharynx
41 Cricothyroid
42 Arch of cricoid cartilage
43 Cricotracheal ligament
44 Trachea
45 Recurrent laryngeal nerve
46 Inferior laryngeal artery
47 Inferior thyroid artery
48 Middle cervical sympathetic ganglion
49 Vagus nerve
50 Scalenus anterior
51 Ventral ramus of fourth cervical nerve
52 Sympathetic trunk
53 Ascending pharyngeal artery
54 Superior laryngeal nerve
55 Superior root of ansa cervicalis
56 Occipital artery
57 Transverse process of atlas
58 Accessory nerve
59 Posterior auricular artery
60 Internal jugular vein
61 Stylohyoid
62 Styloid process
63 Longus capitis

B **The right internal surface** (*after removal of the mucous membrane and pharyngobasilar fascia. The tongue and uvula have been displaced forwards, and the epiglottis backwards*)

64 Sphenoidal sinus
65 Vomer (posterior part of nasal septum)
66 Tensor veli palatini
67 Cartilaginous part of auditory tube
68 Levator veli palatini
69 Soft palate
70 Uvula
71 Palatopharyngeus
72 Salpingopharyngeus
73 Superior constrictor
74 Longus capitis
75 Attachment of pharyngeal raphe to pharyngeal tubercle
76 Middle constrictor
77 Inferior constrictor
78 Piriform fossa
79 Lamina of cricoid cartilage
80 Epiglottis
81 Pharyngeal wall overlying superior horn of thyroid cartilage
82 Greater horn of hyoid bone
83 Stylohyoid ligament
84 Glossopharyngeal nerve
85 Postsulcal part of dorsum of tongue
86 Palatoglossus

● Palatopharyngeus (with salpingopharyngeus joining it) passes downwards *internal* to the superior constrictor.
● Stylopharyngeus passes downwards *between* the superior and middle constrictors.
● Fibres from palatopharyngeus and stylopharyngeus reach the posterior border of the lamina of the thyroid cartilage, and together with the inferior constrictor of the pharynx are important in helping to elevate the *larynx* during swallowing.
● All the muscles of the pharynx are supplied by the pharyngeal plexus except the stylopharyngeus which is supplied by the muscular branch of the glossopharyngeal nerve. The cricopharyngeal part of the inferior constrictor receives an additional supply from the external laryngeal nerve.

● Passing superficial to hyoglossus: the lingual nerve, submandibular duct and hypoglossal nerve.
● Passing deep to the posterior border of hyoglossus: the glossopharyngeal nerve, stylohyoid ligament and lingual artery.

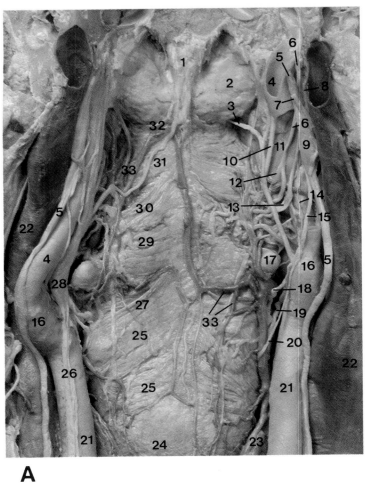

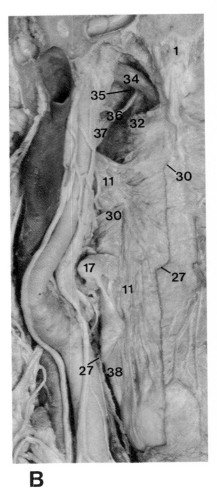

A

B

THE MOUTH, PALATE AND PHARYNX

The pharynx from behind

A From behind *(with the sympathetic trunk and part of the internal carotid artery removed on the right)*

B The left half, from behind *(after removal of the left part of the pharyngobasilar fascia and parts of the middle and inferior constrictors)*

1 Attachment of pharyngeal raphe to pharyngeal tubercle
2 Pharyngobasilar fascia
3 Ascending pharyngeal artery
4 Internal carotid artery
5 Vagus nerve
6 Glossopharyngeal nerve
7 Accessory nerve
8 Hypoglossal nerve
9 Inferior ganglion of vagus nerve
10 Posterior meningeal artery
11 Stylopharyngeus
12 Pharyngeal branch of glossopharyngeal nerve
13 Pharyngeal branch of vagus nerve
14 Vagal branch to carotid body
15 Superior laryngeal branch of vagus nerve
16 Carotid sinus
17 Tip of greater horn of hyoid bone
18 Internal laryngeal nerve
19 Superior thyroid artery
20 External laryngeal nerve
21 Common carotid artery
22 Internal jugular vein
23 Lateral lobe of thyroid gland
24 Cricopharyngeal part ⎫ of inferior
25 Thyropharyngeal part ⎭ constrictor
26 Sympathetic trunk
27 Upper border of inferior constrictor
28 Superior cervical sympathetic ganglion
29 Middle constrictor
30 Upper border of middle constrictor
31 Superior constrictor
32 Upper border of superior constrictor
33 Pharyngeal veins
34 Levator veli palatini
35 Tensor veli palatini
36 Ascending palatine artery
37 Medial pterygoid
38 Posterior border of lamina of thyroid cartilage

● The pharynx extends from the base of the skull to the level of the sixth cervical vertebra, a distance of about 12 cm.
● The nasal part (nasopharynx) extends as far down as the lower border of the soft palate. It contains the opening of the auditory tube and the pharyngeal recess laterally, the pharyngeal tonsil on the posterior wall, and opens anteriorly into the nasal cavity through the posterior nasal apertures (choanae).

● The oral part (oropharynx), between the soft palate and the upper border of the epiglottis, contains the (palatine) tonsil and palatopharyngeal arch in its lateral wall, and opens anteriorly into the mouth through the oropharyngeal isthmus (palatoglossal arches).
● The laryngeal part (laryngopharynx) extends from the upper border of the epiglottis to the lower border of the cricoid cartilage, and is continuous below with the oesophagus. The larynx projects backwards into it, with the piriform fossae on either side of the laryngeal inlet.
● The pharyngobasilar fascia is the thickened submucosa of the pharynx that extends between the upper border of the superior constrictor and the base of the skull.
● The buccopharyngeal fascia (which is very much thinner than the pharyngobasilar fascia) lies on the external surface of the pharyngeal constrictors, and is continued anteriorly on to the outer surface of the buccinator.
● Some of the uppermost fibres of the superior constrictor and of the palatopharyngeus form a muscular band that during swallowing raises a transverse ridge (Passavant's ridge) on the posterior pharyngeal wall which, together with elevation of the soft palate, closes off the nasal part of the pharynx from the oral part.
● The pharyngeal plexuses (of nerves and of veins) are situated mainly on the posterior surface of the middle constrictor.
● The pharyngeal plexus of nerves is formed by the pharyngeal branches of the glossopharyngeal and vagus nerves. The glossopharyngeal component is afferent only; the vagal component is motor to the pharynx and palate as well as containing afferent fibres.

● Glossopharyngeal nerve paralysis:
    No detectable motor disability, as the nerve supplies only one small muscle, stylopharyngeus.
    Loss of taste from the posterior one-third of the tongue, with anaesthesia in the same area and in part of the pharyngeal mucous membrane.

● Vagus and cranial accessory nerve paralysis:
    Paralysis of the soft palate on the affected side (the palate is pulled towards the unaffected side on saying 'Ah').
    Dysphagia (difficulty in swallowing) due to paralysis of pharyngeal muscles.
    Hoarseness of voice due to paralysis of laryngeal muscles.

● Spinal accessory nerve paralysis:
    Paralysis of sternocleidomastoid and trapezius.

● Hypoglossal nerve paralysis:
    Paralysis of the tongue on the affected side (with deviation towards the affected side on protrusion, due to the unopposed action of the intact side).

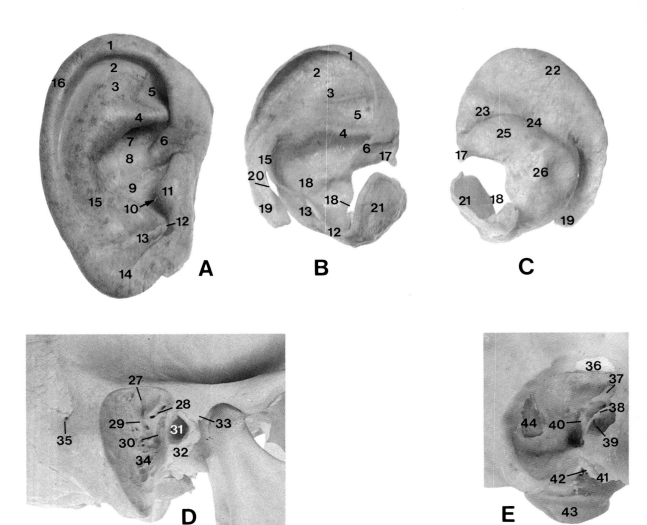

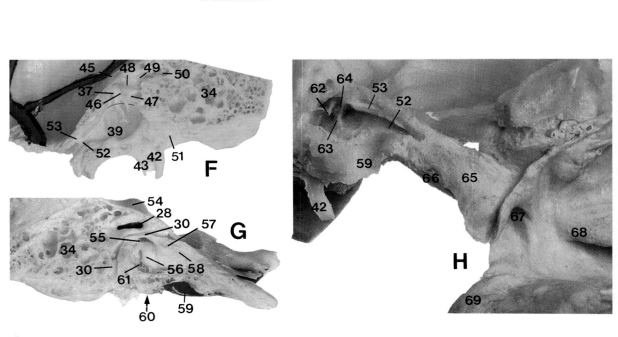

The Ear

The external ear

A Right auricle, from the lateral side
B Right auricular cartilage, from the lateral side
C Right auricular cartilage, from the medial side

1 Helix
2 Scaphoid fossa
3 Upper crus of antihelix
4 Lower crus of antihelix
5 Triangular fossa
6 Crus of helix
7 Cymba conchae
8 Concha
9 Cavum conchae
10 External acoustic meatus
11 Tragus
12 Intertragic notch
13 Antitragus
14 Lobule
15 Antihelix

16 Position of auricular tubercle (if present)
17 Spine of helix
18 Terminal notch
19 Tail of helix
20 Antitragohelicine notch
21 Cartilage of external acoustic meatus
22 Scaphoid eminence
23 Triangular eminence
24 Transverse antihelicine groove
25 Conchal eminence
26 Ponticulus

The middle and internal ear

D Dissection through the right mastoid process (in a dried skull) from the right
E Dissection through the right mastoid process, from the right and behind
F Section through the right temporal bone showing the lateral wall of the middle ear, from the left (with a black bristle indicating the chorda tympani)
G Section through the right temporal bone showing the medial wall of the middle ear, from the right
H The left auditory tube and the lateral wall of the middle ear, and the nasal part of the pharynx, from the right (magnified ×1.5)

27 Anterior
28 Lateral
29 Posterior
} semicircular canal
30 Canal for facial nerve
31 External acoustic meatus
32 Tympanic part of temporal bone
33 Postglenoid tubercle
34 Mastoid air cells
35 Mastoid foramen

36 Dura mater of middle cranial fossa
37 Head of malleus in epitympanic recess
38 Chorda tympani
39 Tympanic membrane
40 Facial nerve
41 Sheath of styloid process
42 Styloid process
43 Occipital condyle
44 Dura mater of sigmoid sinus
45 Tegmen tympani
46 Incudomallear joint
47 Body of incus
48 Epitympanic recess
49 Aditus to mastoid antrum
50 Mastoid antrum
51 Stylomastoid foramen
52 Semicanal for auditory tube
53 Semicanal for tensor tympani
54 Arcuate eminence (overlying anterior semicircular canal)
55 Oval window (fenestra vestibuli)
56 Promontory
57 Trochleariform (cochleariform) process
58 Position of opening of auditory tube
59 Carotid canal
60 Jugular bulb
61 Round window (fenestra cochleae)
62 Incudostapedial joint
63 Handle of malleus
64 Tendon of tensor tympani and 57
65 Medial lamina
66 Lateral lamina
} of cartilaginous part of auditory tube
67 Opening of auditory tube
68 Inferior nasal concha
69 Soft palate

● The external ear consists of the auricle (pinna) and the external acoustic meatus, at the medial end of which lies the tympanic membrane, separating the external ear from the middle ear.

● The middle ear (tympanic cavity) is an irregular space in the temporal bone, lined with mucous membrane, containing the auditory ossicles (malleus, incus and stapes) and filled with air that communicates with the nasopharynx through the auditory tube (Eustachian tube).

● The tympanic cavity consists of the cavity proper and the epitympanic recess.
● The epitympanic recess is the part of the tympanic cavity that projects upwards above the tympanic membrane, and lodges the head of the malleus and the body of the incus. It leads backwards through the aditus into the mastoid antrum, which is an enlarged mastoid air cell.

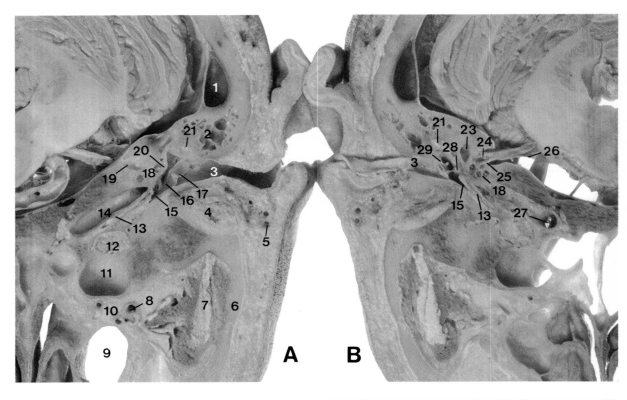

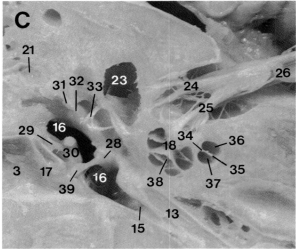

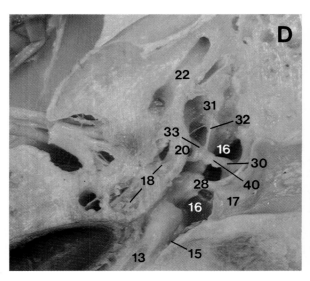

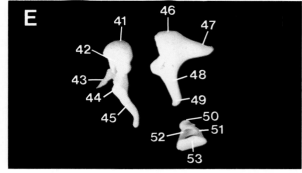

THE EAR

Horizontal section through the external, middle and internal ear

A The lower surface of a section through a left ear, from above
B The upper surface of the same section, from below (*The two sections thus resemble adjacent pages in a book that has been opened up*)
C The central area of B (*magnified ×4*)
D The upper surface of a section through a right ear, from below (*magnified ×4*) (*This section is at a slightly lower level than the section in B and C*)

1 Sigmoid sinus
2 Mastoid air cells
3 External acoustic meatus
4 Intra-articular disc of temporomandibular joint
5 Superficial temporal artery
6 Zygomatic arch
7 Temporalis
8 Maxillary artery
9 Maxillary sinus
10 Pterygopalatine fossa
11 Sphenoidal sinus
12 Cavernous sinus
13 Semicanal with tensor tympani
14 Internal carotid artery in carotid canal
15 Opening of auditory tube
16 Cavity of middle ear
17 Tympanic membrane
18 Cochlea
19 Floor of internal acoustic meatus
20 Promontory
21 Facial nerve
22 Posterior semicircular canal
23 Vestibular part of osseous labyrinth
24 Vestibular part ⎱ of vestibulocochlear nerve
25 Cochlear part ⎰ in internal acoustic meatus
26 Labyrinthine artery
27 Internal carotid artery in foramen lacerum
28 Tendon of tensor tympani and trochleariform (cochleariform) process
29 Chorda tympani
30 Long limb of incus
31 Pyramid
32 Stapedius
33 Stapes
34 Osseous spiral lamina
35 Basilar membrane
36 Scala tympani
37 Scala vestibuli
38 Modiolus
39 Handle of malleus
40 Incudostapedial joint

E The disarticulated auditory ossicles of the right ear (*magnified ×4*)

41 Head ⎫
42 Neck ⎬
43 Anterior process ⎬ of malleus
44 Lateral process ⎬
45 Handle ⎭
46 Body ⎫
47 Short limb ⎬ of incus
48 Long limb ⎬
49 Lenticular process ⎭
50 Head ⎫
51 Posterior limb ⎬
52 Anterior limb ⎬ of stapes
53 Base (footplate) ⎭

● For the genicular ganglion of the facial nerve see page 166.

● Features of the walls of the middle ear:
Lateral wall – the tympanic membrane, part of the petrotympanic fissure, the anterior and posterior canaliculi for the chorda tympani.
Medial wall (from above downwards) – the prominence due to the lateral semicircular canal, the prominence due to the canal for the facial nerve, the promontory (due to the first turn of the cochlea), with the oval window (fenestra vestibuli) occupied by the footplate of the stapes *above and behind* the promontory, and the round window (fenestra cochleae) occupied by the secondary tympanic membrane *below and behind* the promontory.
Roof – the tegmen tympani (part of the petrous part of the temporal bone).
Floor – above the superior bulb of the internal jugular vein, with the canaliculus for the tympanic branch of the glossopharyngeal nerve.
Anterior wall – the carotid canal with (laterally) the openings of the semicanals for the tensor tympani and the auditory tube.
Posterior wall – the aditus to the mastoid antrum, the pyramid (with stapedius emerging) in front of the vertical part of the canal for the facial nerve, and the fossa for the incus.

● The internal ear consists of the osseous labyrinth and the membranous labyrinth.
● The osseous labyrinth (within the temporal bone) consists of the vestibule, the semicircular canals and the cochlea.
● The membranous labyrinth is inside the bony labyrinth and consists of the utricle and saccule (within the vestibule), the semicircular ducts (within the semicircular canals), and the duct of the cochlea (within the cochlea).
● The membranous labyrinth contains endolymph and is separated from the bony labyrinth by perilymph. These two fluids do not communicate with one another, but the perilymph probably communicates with the cerebrospinal fluid in the subarachnoid space via the cochlear canaliculus.

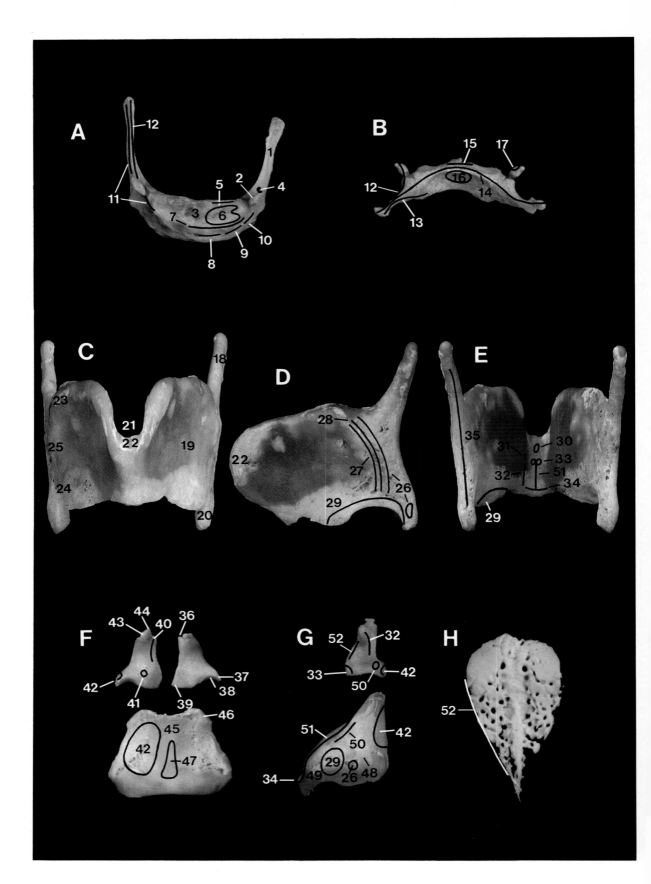

152

The Larynx

The hyoid bone and cartilages of the larynx

The hyoid bone

A From above and in front, with attachments
B From behind, with attachments

1 Greater horn
2 Lesser horn
3 Body
4 Stylohyoid ligament
5 Genioglossus
6 Geniohyoid
7 Mylohyoid
8 Sternohyoid
9 Omohyoid
10 Stylohyoid
11 Hyoglossus
12 Middle constrictor
13 Thyrohyoid
14 Thyrohyoid membrane
15 Hyoepiglottic ligament
16 Bursa
17 Chondroglossus

The thyroid cartilage

C From the front
D From the left, with attachments
E From behind, with attachments

18 Superior horn
19 Lamina
20 Inferior horn
21 Thyroid notch
22 Laryngeal prominence (Adam's apple)
23 Superior ⎫
24 Inferior ⎬ tubercle
25 Oblique line
26 Inferior constrictor
27 Sternothyroid
28 Thyrohyoid
29 Cricothyroid
30 Thyro-epiglottic ligament
31 Thyro-epiglottic muscle
32 Thyro-arytenoid
33 Vocal ligament
34 Conus elasticus
35 Stylopharyngeus and palatopharyngeus

The cricoid and arytenoid cartilages

F From behind, with attachments
G From the left, with attachments

36 Apex ⎫
37 Muscular process ⎬ of arytenoid cartilage
38 Articular surface ⎬
39 Vocal process ⎭
40 Transverse arytenoid
41 Oblique arytenoid
42 Posterior crico-arytenoid
43 Corniculate cartilage
44 Cuneiform cartilage
45 Lamina of cricoid cartilage
46 Articular surface for arytenoid cartilage
47 Tendon of oesophagus
48 Articular surface for inferior horn of thyroid cartilage
49 Arch
50 Lateral crico-arytenoid
51 Cricothyroid ligament
52 Quadrangular membrane

The epiglottic cartilage

H From behind

● The hyoid bone consists of a body with greater and lesser horns on each side.
● The thyroid cartilage consists of two laminae united anteriorly and with superior and inferior horns posteriorly. The gap above the united laminae is the thyroid notch which is bounded below by the laryngeal prominence (Adam's apple). The angle between the laminae is more acute in males than in females, in whom the prominence is less obvious.
● The cricoid cartilage is shaped like a signet ring, with an arch anteriorly and a lamina at the back.
● The paired arytenoid cartilages have the shape of a three-sided pyramid, with at the base an (anterior) vocal process to which the vocal ligament is attached and a (lateral) muscular process to which the posterior and lateral crico-arytenoid muscles are attached.
● The thyroid, cricoid and almost all of the arytenoid cartilages are composed of hyaline cartilage and may undergo some degree of calcification (becoming visible on radiographs).
● The apex of the arytenoid cartilage is composed of elastic fibro-cartilage, like the epiglottic cartilage (which is leaf-shaped with numerous pits or perforations) and the corniculate and cuneiform cartilages (which are like small pips or rice grains). The triticeal cartilages are very small nodules that are often found in the posterior margin of the thyrohyoid membrane.

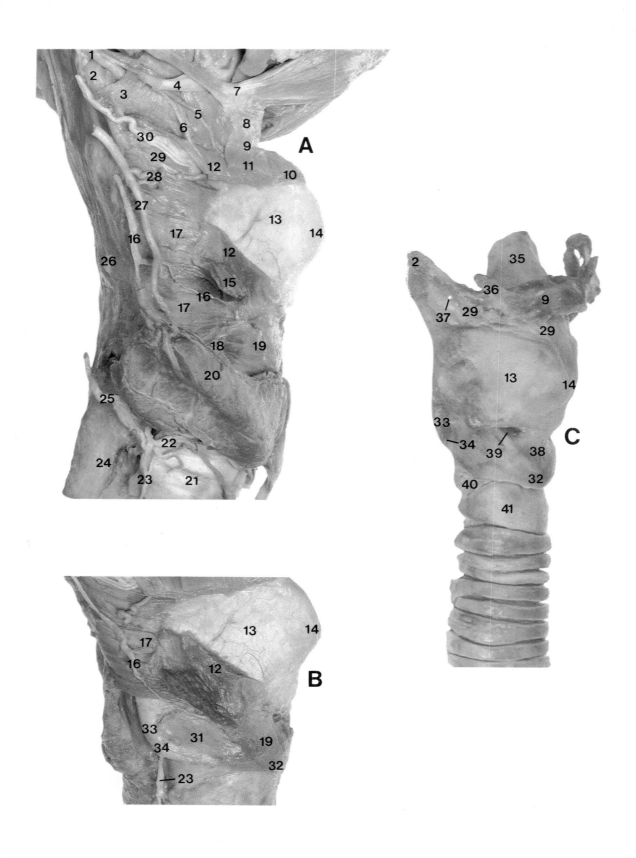

154

THE LARYNX

The larynx with the pharynx, hyoid bone and trachea

A From the right *(with the lateral lobe of the thyroid gland displaced slightly backwards)*
B After removal of the thyroid gland and part of the inferior constrictor
C From the front and the right after removal of muscles

(For a view of the inlet (aditus) of the larynx see page 139)

(For a view of the inlet (aditus) of the larynx see page 139)

1 Lingual artery
2 Tip of greater horn of hyoid bone
3 Hyoglossus
4 Hypoglossal nerve
5 Suprahyoid artery
6 Nerve to thyrohyoid
7 Tendon of digastric
8 Digastric sling
9 Body of hyoid bone
10 Sternohyoid
11 Superior belly of omohyoid
12 Thyrohyoid
13 Lamina of thyroid cartilage
14 Laryngeal prominence
15 Sternothyroid
16 External laryngeal nerve
17 Inferior constrictor
18 Tendinous band
19 Cricothyroid (straight part)
20 Lateral lobe of thyroid gland
21 Trachea
22 Inferior laryngeal artery
23 Recurrent laryngeal nerve
24 Oesophagus
25 Inferior thyroid artery
26 Posterior pharyngeal wall
27 Superior thyroid artery
28 Superior laryngeal artery
29 Thyrohyoid membrane
30 Internal laryngeal nerve
31 Cricothyroid (oblique part)
32 Arch of cricoid cartilage
33 Inferior horn of thyroid cartilage
34 Cricothyroid joint
35 Epiglottis
36 Lesser horn of hyoid bone
37 Aperture for internal laryngeal nerve and superior laryngeal artery
38 Conus elasticus (central part of cricothyroid membrane)
39 Cricothyroid membrane (lateral part)
40 Cricotracheal ligament
41 First tracheal ring (unusually large)

● The intrinsic muscles of the larynx are supplied by the recurrent laryngeal nerve, except the cricothyroid which is supplied by the external laryngeal nerve.
● The mucous membrane of the larynx *above* the level of the vocal folds is supplied by the internal laryngeal nerve, and *below* the vocal folds by the recurrent laryngeal nerve.
● The internal laryngeal nerve enters the *pharynx* by piercing the thyrohoid membrane, and from there fibres spread into the larynx.
● The recurrent laryngeal nerve lies immediately behind the cricothyroid joint, and enters the larynx by passing deep to the lower border of the inferior constrictor of the pharynx.

● In *complete* paralysis of the recurrent laryngeal nerve, there is permanent hoarseness of the voice, and the affected vocal cord assumes the 'cadaveric' position, midway between full abduction and adduction.

● In *incomplete* paralysis of the recurrent laryngeal nerve, the affected cord takes up the adducted position.

● In paralysis of the external laryngeal nerve there may be no detectable abnormality. If there is any, there is some hoarseness due to loss of tension in the affected cord from the paralysed cricothyroid, but the hoarseness will disappear due to hypertrophy of the opposite cricothyroid.

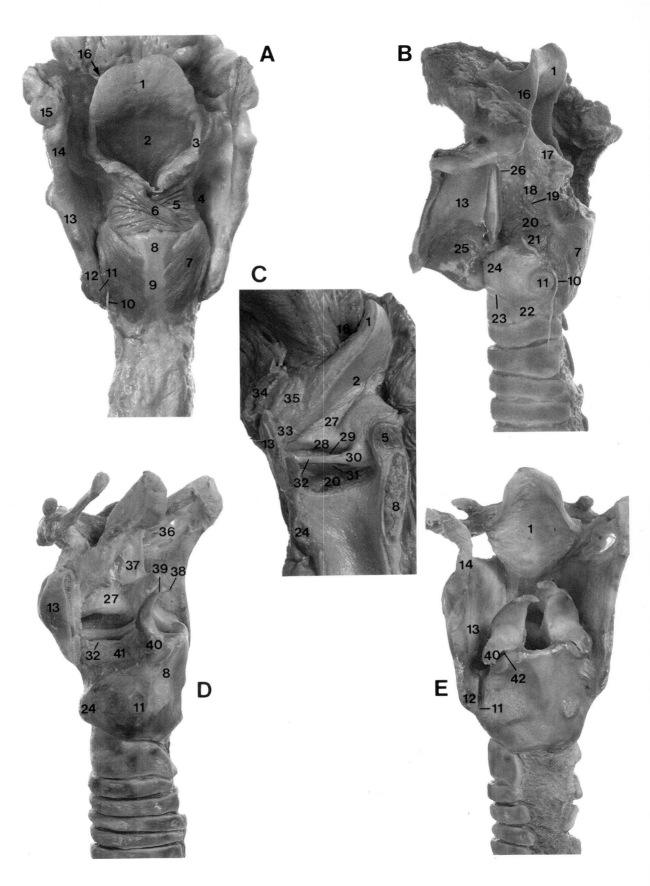

THE LARYNX

The muscles, ligaments and membranes

A From behind
B From the left *(after reflecting the thyroid lamina forwards)*
C The internal surface of the right half *(after removal of most of the cricothyroid ligament and the overlying mucous membrane)*
D From the left *(after resecting most of the left thyroid lamina)*
E From behind *(after removal of muscles in an asymmetric specimen)*

1 Epiglottis
2 Vestibule
3 Aryepiglottic fold
4 Piriform fossa
5 Transverse arytenoid
6 Oblique arytenoid
7 Posterior crico-arytenoid
8 Lamina of cricoid cartilage
9 Site of attachment of oesophageal tendon
10 Recurrent laryngeal nerve
11 Cricothyroid joint
12 Inferior horn ⎫
13 Lamina ⎬ of thyroid cartilage
14 Superior horn ⎭
15 Greater horn of hyoid bone
16 Vallecula
17 Aryepiglottic muscle
18 Thyro-epiglottic muscle
19 Superior thyro-arytenoid
20 Thyro-arytenoid
21 Lateral crico-arytenoid
22 First tracheal ring
23 Cricotracheal ligament
24 Arch of cricoid cartilage
25 Cricothyroid
26 Internal laryngeal nerve
27 Vestibule and mucous membrane overlying quadrangular membrane
28 Vestibular fold
29 Ventricle of larynx
30 Vocal process of arytenoid cartilage
31 Vocalis part of thyro-arytenoid
32 Vocal ligament
33 Thyro-epiglottic ligament
34 Body of hyoid bone
35 Hyo-epiglottic ligament
36 Thyrohyoid membrane
37 Quadrangular membrane
38 Cuneiform cartilage
39 Corniculate cartilage
40 Muscular process of arytenoid cartilage
41 Cricothyroid ligament
42 Crico-arytenoid joint

● The central part of the cricothyroid ligament is usually known as the conus elasticus (although some texts use this term for the whole ligament). The lateral part of the cricothyroid ligament is sometimes known as the cricovocal membrane.
● The upper (free) margin of the cricothyroid ligament is slightly thickened to form the vocal ligament. Covered by mucous membrane it becomes the vocal fold (vocal cord), and is attached anteriorly to the lamina of the thyroid cartilage adjacent to the midline, and posteriorly to the vocal process of the arytenoid cartilage.
● The lower margin of the cricothyroid ligament is not free but attached to the upper border of the lamina and arch of the cricoid cartilage.

● The quadrangular membrane (a very thin sheet of connective tissue which has been artificially thickened for emphasis in D) passes between the lateral side of the arytenoid cartilage (which is relatively short) to the lateral edge of the epiglottic cartilage (which is relatively long). The membrane is thus an irregular quadrilateral in shape and not rectangular.
● The upper (free) margin of the quadrangular membrane is covered by mucous membrane to form the aryepiglottic fold.
● The lower (free) margin of the quadrangular membrane is covered by mucous membrane to form the vestibular fold (false vocal cord).

● The slit-like space between the vestibular and vocal folds is the ventricle (or sinus) of the larynx, and is continuous with the saccule, a small pouch of mucous membrane that extends upwards for a few millimetres at the anterior part of the ventricle between the vestibular fold and the inner surface of the thyroid lamina. Mucous secretion from glands in the saccule lubricates the vocal folds.

● The posterior crico-arytenoid is commonly accepted to be the one muscle that can abduct the vocal fold (open the glottis).
● The lateral crico-arytenoid and the transverse and oblique arytenoids adduct the vocal fold (close the glottis).
● The cricothyroid lengthens (and may increase tension in) the vocal fold.

The Cranial Cavity

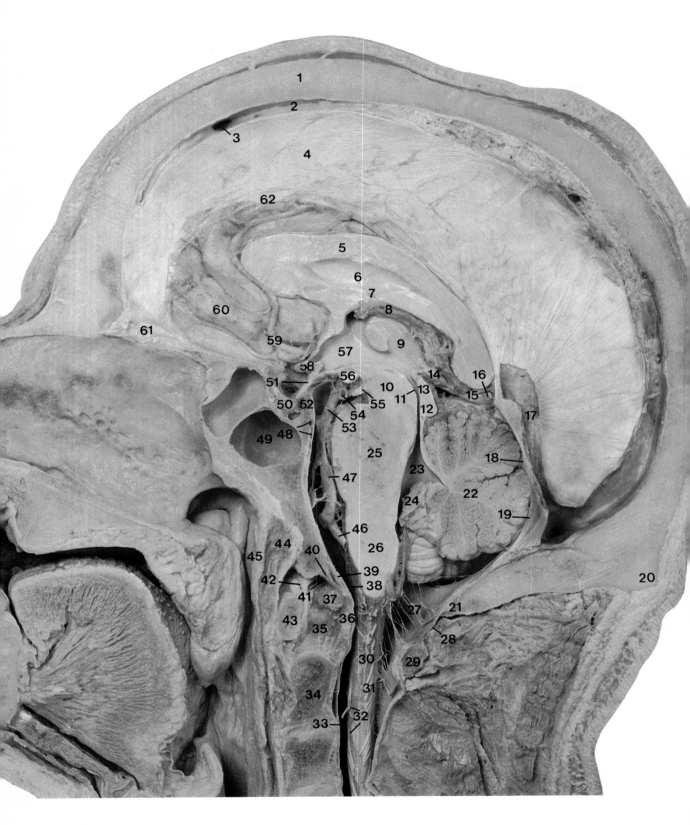

THE CRANIAL CAVITY

The cranial cavity, brain and meninges

The right half of a sagittal section, slightly to the left of the midline

1 Vault of skull
2 Superior sagittal sinus
3 Aperture of a superior cerebral vein
4 Falx cerebri
5 Corpus callosum
6 Septum pellucidum
7 Body of fornix
8 Choroid plexus of third ventricle
9 Thalamus and third ventricle
10 Midbrain
11 Aqueduct of midbrain
12 Inferior colliculus
13 Superior colliculus
14 Pineal body
15 Great cerebral vein
16 Basal vein
17 Straight sinus
18 Tentorium cerebelli
19 Falx cerebelli
20 External occipital protuberance
21 Posterior margin of foramen magnum
22 Cerebellum
23 Fourth ventricle
24 Choroid plexus of fourth ventricle
25 Pons
26 Medulla oblongata
27 Filaments of arachnoid mater in cerebellomedullary cistern (cisterna magna)
28 Posterior atlanto-occipital membrane and overlying dura mater
29 Posterior arch of atlas
30 Spinal cord (spinal medulla)
31 Dorsal rootlets ⎫
32 Ventral rootlets ⎭ of spinal nerves
33 Spinal subarachnoid space
34 Body of axis
35 Dens of axis (left side)
36 Transverse ligament of atlas
37 Alar ligament
38 Dura mater
39 Tectorial membrane
40 Superior longitudinal band of cruciform ligament
41 Apical ligament
42 Anterior atlanto-occipital membrane
43 Anterior arch of atlas
44 Longus capitis
45 Posterior pharyngeal wall
46 Vertebral artery
47 Basilar artery
48 Basilar sinus
49 Sphenoidal sinus
50 Pituitary gland
51 Pituitary stalk
52 Dorsum sellae
53 Superior cerebellar artery
54 Posterior cerebral artery
55 Oculomotor nerve
56 Mamillary body
57 Hypothalamus
58 Optic chiasma
59 Anterior cerebral artery
60 Arachnoid mater overlying medial surface of cerebral hemisphere
61 Crista galli
62 Lower border of falx cerebri and inferior sagittal sinus

● The dura mater is sometimes known as the pachymeninx; the arachnoid and pia mater together constitute the leptomeninges.

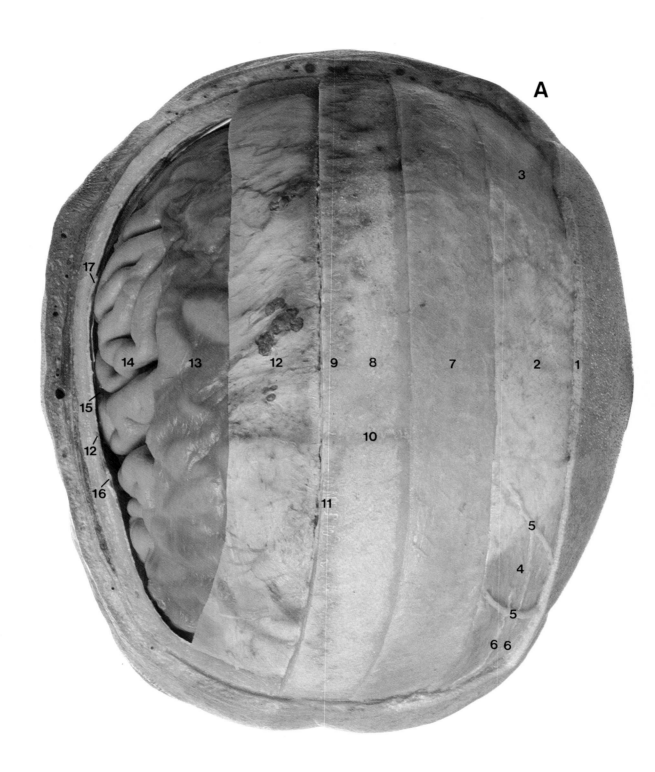

A

THE CRANIAL CAVITY

The cranial cavity and its coverings, from above

A **Layered dissection, from above**
B **Cerebral dura mater, from the right** (*The dotted circle indicates the position of pterion*)

 1 Skin and dense subcutaneous tissue
 2 Epicranial aponeurosis (galea aponeurotica)
 3 Occipital belly ⎫
 4 Frontal belly ⎬ of occipitofrontalis
 5 Branches of superficial temporal artery
 6 Branches of supra-orbital nerve
 7 Loose connective tissue and pericranium
 8 Bone of cranial vault
 9 Sagittal suture
10 Coronal suture
11 Frontal (metopic) suture
12 Dura mater
13 Arachnoid mater
14 Cerebral hemisphere covered by pia mater
15 Subarachnoid space
16 Frontal branch ⎫
17 Parietal branch ⎬ of middle meningeal artery
18 Scalp
19 Arachnoid granulation

● The scalp consists of five layers:
   the skin
   dense connective tissue
   the epicranial aponeurosis and the occipitofrontalis
      muscle
   loose connective tissue
   the pericranium (periosteum on the outer surface of the
      cranial vault)

● The meninges comprise the dura mater, arachnoid mater and pia mater.

● The dura mater has cerebral and spinal parts.
● The cerebral part of the dura mater lines the inside of the skull and consists of an outer endosteal layer (corresponding to periosteum) which ends at the foramen magnum, and an inner meningeal layer which forms sheaths for the cranial nerves as they pass out through skull foramina, and also forms four processes – the falx cerebri, tentorium cerebelli, falx cerebelli and diaphragma sellae.
● The venous sinuses of the dura mater lie between the endosteal and meningeal layers and can be divided into two groups:

Posterosuperior	*Antero-inferior*
Superior sagittal	Cavernous (paired)
Inferior sagittal	Intercavernous
Straight	Sphenoparietal (paired)
Transverse (paired)	Superior petrosal (paired)
Sigmoid (paired)	Inferior petrosal (paired)
Petrosquamous (paired)	Basilar
Occipital	Middle meningeal veins (paired)

● The spinal part of the dura mater corresponds to the meningeal layer of the cerebral part and forms a sheath for the spinal cord within the vertebral canal.

● The arachnoid mater lies inside the dura mater separated from it by the subdural space which is merely a capillary interval.

● The pia mater adheres intimately to the surface of the brain and spinal cord, and is separated from the arachnoid mater by the subarachnoid space which contains the cerebrospinal fluid. The pia mater forms the denticulate ligament, filum terminale and subarachnoid septum.

● The middle meningeal artery does *not* supply the brain; it lies between the dura mater and the skull.

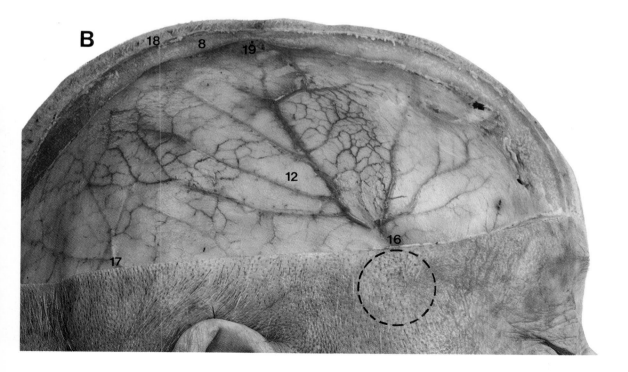

B

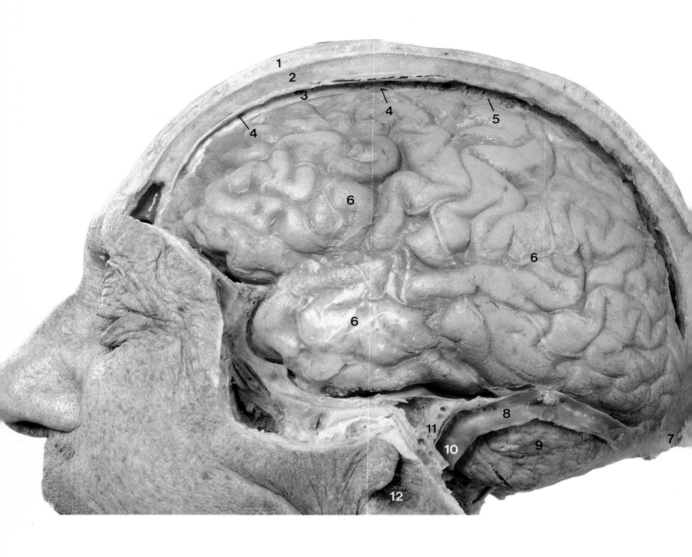

THE CRANIAL CAVITY

The brain in situ

From the left *(after removal of part of the skull and dura mater)*

1 Scalp
2 Cranial vault
3 Superior sagittal sinus
4 Openings of superior cerebral veins
5 Arachnoid granulations
6 Vessels and arachnoid mater overlying cerebral hemisphere
7 External occipital protuberance
8 Transverse sinus
9 Cerebellar hemisphere
10 Sigmoid sinus
11 Mastoid air cells
12 External acoustic meatus

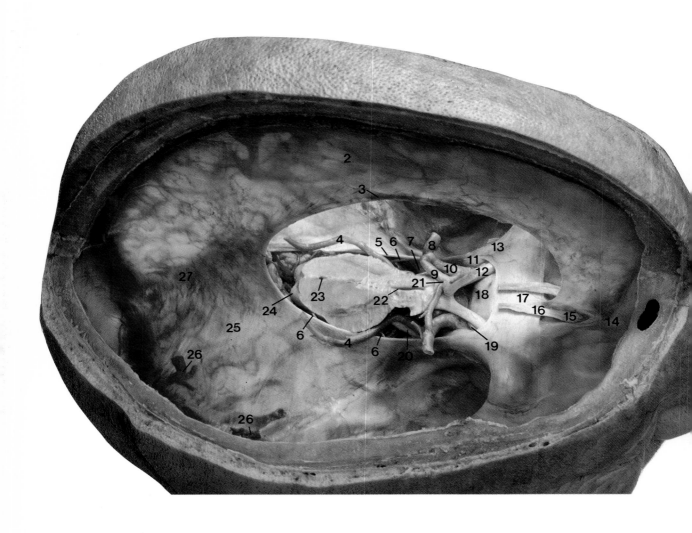

THE CRANIAL CAVITY

The falx cerebri and tentorium cerebelli

From the right and above, with part of the brainstem in situ

 1 Superior sagittal sinus
 2 Falx cerebri
 3 Inferior sagittal sinus
 4 Posterior cerebral artery
 5 Free margin of tentorium cerebelli
 6 Trochlear nerve
 7 Attached margin of tentorium cerebelli and superior margin of petrous part of temporal bone with superior petrosal sinus
 8 Middle cerebral artery
 9 Anterior cerebral artery
10 Internal carotid artery
11 Anterior clinoid process
12 Optic nerve
13 Posterior margin of lesser wing of sphenoid bone and sphenoparietal sinus
14 Crista galli
15 Olfactory bulb
16 Olfactory tract
17 Jugum of sphenoid bone
18 Prechiasmatic groove
19 Ophthalmic artery
20 Oculomotor nerve
21 Anterior communicating artery
22 Third ventricle
23 Aqueduct of midbrain
24 Inferior colliculus
25 Tentorium cerebelli
26 Inferior cerebral veins
27 Straight sinus in junction of **2** and **25**

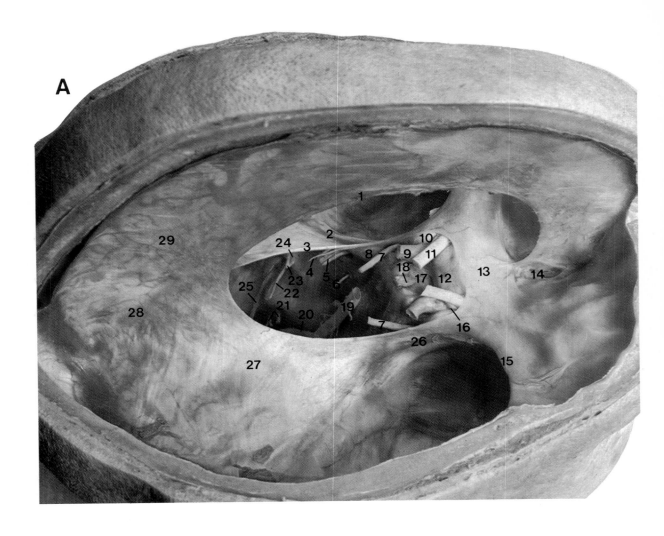

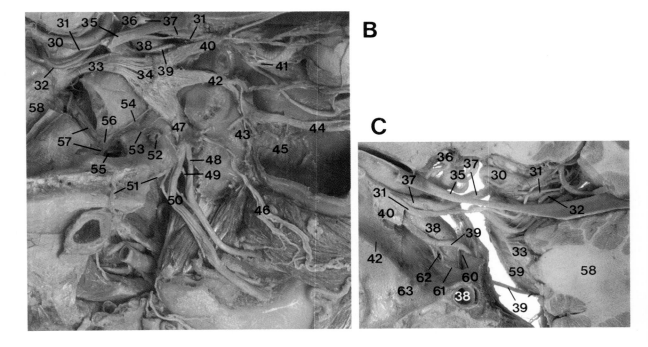

THE CRANIAL CAVITY

The falx cerebri, tentorium cerebelli and cavernous sinus

A The falx and tentorium, from the right, above and behind, with the brainstem removed

 1 Inferior margin of falx cerebri and inferior sagittal sinus
 2 Attached margin of tentorium cerebelli and superior petrosal sinus
 3 Free margin of tentorium cerebelli
 4 Trochlear nerve
 5 Trigeminal nerve
 6 Abducent nerve
 7 Oculomotor nerve
 8 Posterior clinoid process
 9 Internal carotid artery
10 Anterior clinoid process
11 Optic nerve
12 Prechiasmatic groove
13 Jugum of sphenoid bone
14 Cribriform plate of ethmoid bone
15 Posterior margin of lesser wing of sphenoid bone and sphenoparietal sinus
16 Ophthalmic artery
17 Diaphragma sellae
18 Pituitary stalk
19 Basilar artery
20 Left vertebral artery
21 Hypoglossal nerve
22 Roots of glossopharyngeal, vagus and cranial part of accessory nerves
23 Vestibulocochlear nerve
24 Facial nerve
25 Spinal root of·accessory nerve
26 Cavernous sinus
27 Tentorium cerebelli
28 Straight sinus in junction between **27** and **29**
29 Falx cerebri

The cavernous sinus

B The right cavernous sinus, with the trigeminal ganglion and the genicular ganglion of the facial nerve, from the right and above (*after extensive skull dissection*)

C The left cavernous sinus, from the left (*dissected in a sagittal section of the head through the plane of the foramen ovale*)

30 Posterior cerebral artery
31 Trochlear nerve
32 Superior cerebellar artery
33 Trigeminal nerve
34 Trigeminal ganglion
35 Free margin of tentorium cerebelli
36 Middle cerebral artery
37 Oculomotor nerve
38 Internal carotid artery
39 Abducent nerve
40 Ophthalmic nerve entering superior orbital fissure
41 Ciliary ganglion
42 Maxillary nerve in foramen rotundum
43 Posterior superior alveolar nerve
44 Infra-orbital nerve
45 Maxillary sinus
46 Buccal nerve
47 Mandibular nerve in foramen ovale
48 Lingual nerve
49 Chorda tympani
50 Inferior alveolar nerve
51 Auriculotemporal nerve
52 Middle meningeal artery in foramen spinosum
53 Lesser petrosal nerve
54 Greater petrosal nerve
55 Middle ear (tympanic cavity)
56 Genicular ganglion of facial nerve
57 Facial nerve
58 Cerebellum
59 Pons
60 Apex of petrous part of temporal bone
61 Upper margin of foramen lacerum
62 Sympathetic plexus (internal carotid nerve)
63 Foramen ovale

● The cavernous sinus contains the internal carotid artery with its sympathetic plexus, and with the abducent nerve lying on the lateral side of the artery. The oculomotor, trochlear, ophthalmic and maxillary nerves are described as lying in the lateral wall of the sinus.

● The trigeminal ganglion lies in the trigeminal cave of dura mater, on the trigeminal impression at the apex of the petrous part of the temporal bone.

● The facial nerve enters the internal acoustic meatus and runs laterally in the facial canal above the vestibule to the genicular ganglion in the medial wall of the epitympanic recess. The nerve then takes a right-angled turn backwards in the medial wall of the middle ear above the promontory, passes downwards in the medial wall of the aditus to the mastoid antrum, and finally emerges through the stylomastoid foramen. For details of the middle ear see pages 148–151.

● The greater petrosal nerve is joined by the deep petrosal nerve (sympathetic fibres from the plexus round the internal carotid artery) within the foramen lacerum to become the nerve of the pterygoid canal.

● After emerging from the brainstem between the pons and the pyramid, the abducent nerve runs forwards and slightly upwards and laterally through the cisterna pontis to pierce the dura mater on the clivus. The nerve continues upwards beneath the dura to bend forwards over the tip of the apex of the petrous part of the temporal bone and beneath the petrosphenoidal ligament to enter the cavernous sinus. The nerve can be damaged by fractures of the skull that involve the petrous temporal or clivus or by stretching if the brainstem is forced downwards. Displacement of the midbrain may also damage the oculomotor and trochlear nerves.

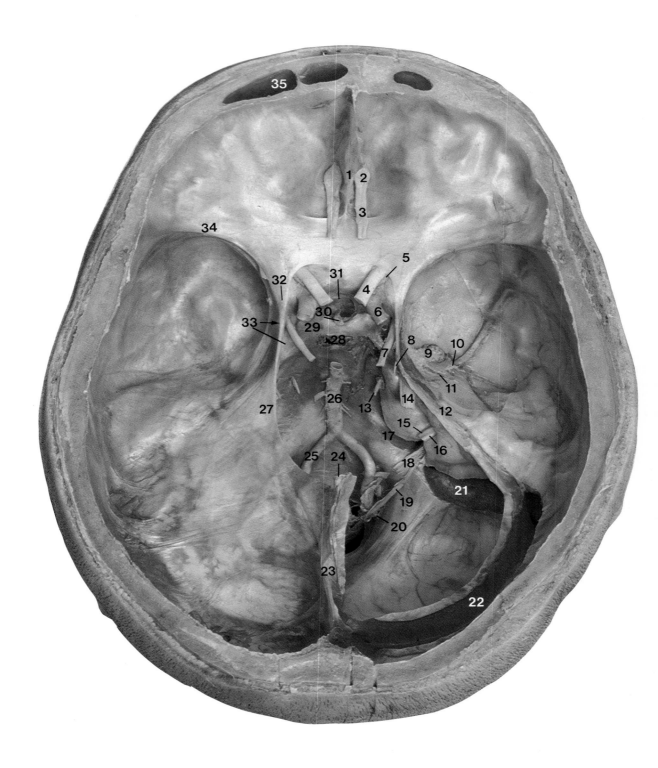

THE CRANIAL CAVITY

The cranial fossae

From above and behind, with the right half of the tentorium cerebelli removed

1 Falx cerebri attached to crista galli
2 Olfactory bulb
3 Olfactory tract
4 Optic nerve
5 Ophthalmic artery
6 Internal carotid artery
7 Oculomotor nerve
8 Trochlear nerve
9 Mandibular nerve and foramen ovale
10 Middle meningeal artery and foramen spinosum
11 Groove for greater petrosal nerve
12 Superior petrosal sinus and cut edges of attached margin of tentorium cerebelli
13 Abducent nerve
14 Trigeminal nerve
15 Facial nerve
16 Vestibulocochlear nerve
17 Inferior petrosal sinus
18 Roots of glossopharyngeal, vagus and cranial part of accessory nerves
19 Spinal root of accessory nerve
20 Hypoglossal nerve
21 Sigmoid sinus
22 Transverse sinus
23 Straight sinus at junction of falx cerebri and tentorium cerebelli
24 Great cerebral vein
25 Vertebral artery
26 Basilar artery
27 Free margin of tentorium cerebelli
28 Upper part of basilar plexus
29 Posterior clinoid process
30 Pituitary stalk
31 Diaphragm sellae
32 Anterior clinoid process
33 Cavernous sinus
34 Posterior margin of lesser wing of sphenoid bone and sphenoparietal sinus
35 Frontal sinus

● For further details of the cranial fossae see pages 64–67.

● The tentorium cerebelli forms the roof of the posterior cranial fossa; the anterior and middle cranial fossae have no defined upper boundary.

● The anterior cranial fossa contains:
the frontal lobes of the cerebral hemispheres
the olfactory nerves, olfactory bulbs and olfactory tracts
the anterior ethmoidal nerve and vessels

● The middle cranial fossa contains *in its median part*:
the pituitary gland
the optic nerves and optic chiasma
the intercavernous sinus
and *in its lateral parts*:
the cavernous sinus containing the internal carotid artery
and its sympathetic nerve plexus, the oculomotor,
trochlear, abducent, ophthalmic and maxillary nerves
the sphenoparietal and superior petrosal sinuses
the trigeminal ganglion and mandibular nerve
the greater and lesser petrosal nerves
the middle meningeal and accessory meningeal vessels, and
meningeal branches of the ascending pharyngeal,
ophthalmic and lacrimal arteries
the temporal lobes of the cerebral hemispheres

● The posterior cranial fossa contains:
the lowest part of the midbrain, the pons, medulla
oblongata and cerebellum
the vertebral and basilar arteries and their branches, and
meningeal branches of the ascending pharyngeal and
occipital arteries
the inferior petrosal, basilar and occipital sinuses, with the
straight, sigmoid and superior petrosal sinuses in the
tentorium cerebelli that forms the roof
the trigeminal, abducent, facial, vestibulocochlear,
glossopharyngeal, vagus, accessory and hypoglossal
nerves (i.e. the fifth to twelfth cranial nerves), and
meningeal branches of upper cervical nerves
the falx cerebelli

● The posterior (lower) end of the superior sagittal sinus is known as the confluence of the sinuses, where there is communication with the straight and occipital sinuses and the transverse sinuses of both sides.

The Brain

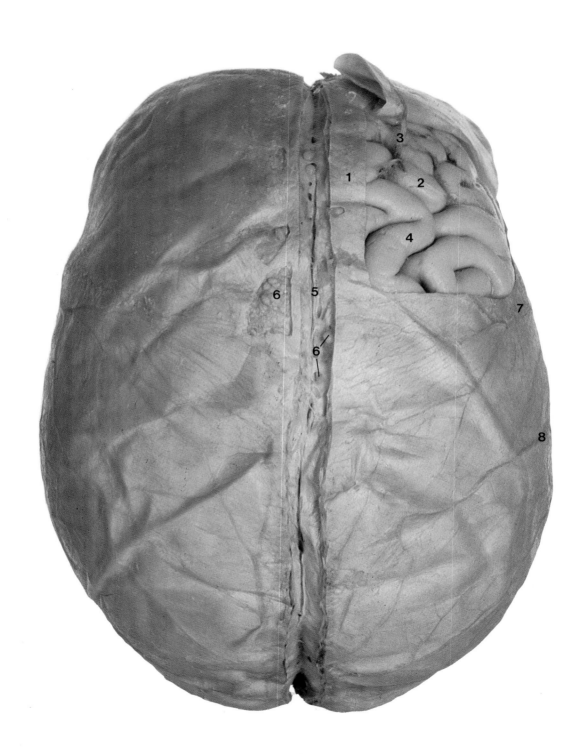

THE BRAIN

The brain within the meninges

From above *(with windows in the dura mater and arachnoid mater)*

1 Dura mater
2 Arachnoid mater
3 A superior cerebral vein
4 Cerebral hemisphere (and pia mater)
5 Superior sagittal sinus
6 Arachnoid granulations
7 Frontal branch ⎫
8 Parietal branch ⎬ of middle meningeal artery

● The central nervous system consists of the brain and the spinal cord (properly called the spinal medulla).

● The brain consists of:
  the hindbrain (rhombencephalon) comprising the medulla oblongata (myelencephalon), the pons (metencephalon) and the cerebellum.
  the midbrain (mesencephalon).
  the forebrain (prosencephalon) comprising the diencephalon (structures surrounding the third ventricle) and the cerebral hemispheres (telencephalon).

● The brainstem consists of the midbrain, pons and medulla oblongata.

● The peripheral nervous system consists of the cranial nerves (12 pairs), the spinal nerves (31 pairs), and the autonomic system of nerves, together with all their associated ganglia.

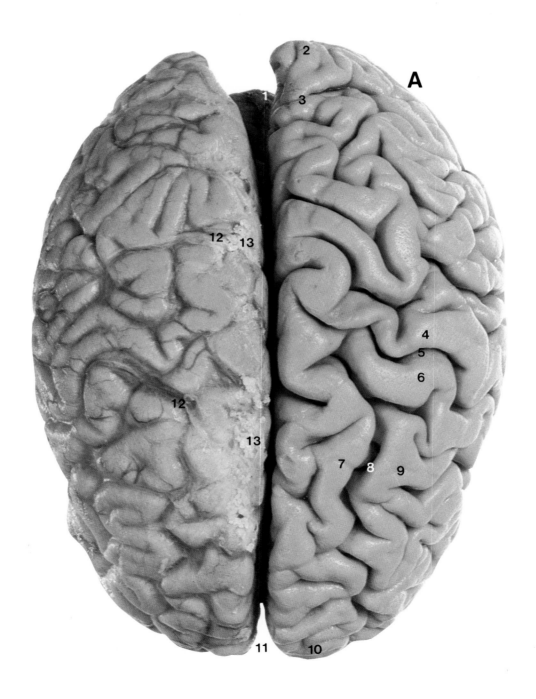

THE BRAIN

The cerebral hemispheres and cerebellum

A From above *(with the arachnoid mater removed from the left cerebral hemisphere)*
B From behind

1 Cerebellum
2 Occipital pole
3 Parieto-occipital sulcus
4 Postcentral gyrus
5 Central sulcus
6 Precentral gyrus
7 Superior frontal gyrus
8 Superior frontal sulcus
9 Middle frontal gyrus
10 Frontal pole
11 Longitudinal fissure
12 Superior cerebral veins
13 Arachnoid granulations
14 Cerebellar hemisphere
15 Arachnoid mater of cerebellomedullary cistern
  (cisterna magna)

● The cerebral cortex (composed of grey matter) is thrown into broad convoluted folds known as gyri; the spaces between the folds are the sulci.

● The cerebellar cortex is thrown into narrow closely-packed folds known as folia.

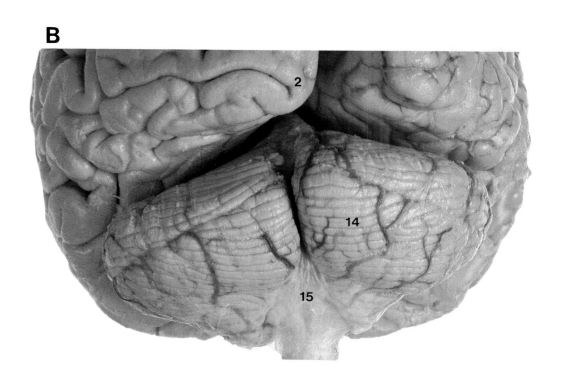

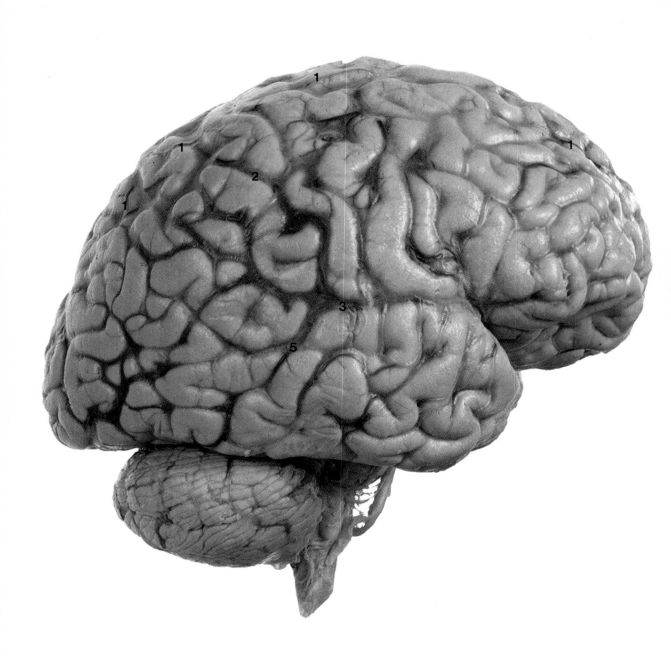

THE BRAIN

The external cerebral veins

From the right *(with the arachnoid mater intact)*

1 Superior cerebral veins
2 Superior anastomotic vein
3 Superficial middle cerebral vein overlying
    posterior ramus of lateral sulcus
4 Inferior cerebral veins
5 Inferior anastomotic vein

● The superior cerebral veins (8 to 12) drain into the superior sagittal sinus, the more posterior veins entering obliquely forwards (against the normal current in the sinus).

● The superficial middle cerebral vein runs forwards along the surface of the lateral sulcus and drains into the cavernous sinus.

● The inferior cerebral veins are small. Those under the frontal lobe join superior cerebral veins and drain into the superior sagittal sinus; from the temporal lobe they drain into the cavernous, superior petrosal and transverse sinuses.

● The superior anastomotic vein runs upwards and backwards from the superficial middle cerebral vein to the superior sagittal sinus, and the inferior anastomotic vein downwards and backwards to the transverse sinus.

● The internal cerebral vein is formed by the union of the thalamostriate and choroidal veins (with some smaller adjacent veins), and runs backwards in the tela choroidea of the roof of the third ventricle, to unite with its fellow beneath the splenium of the corpus callosum to form the great cerebral vein.

● The basal vein, formed by the union of the anterior cerebral vein (which accompanies the artery of the same name), the deep middle cerebral vein (from the insula), and the striate veins (from the anterior perforated substance), passes backwards round the lateral side of the cerebral peduncle to join the great cerebral vein.

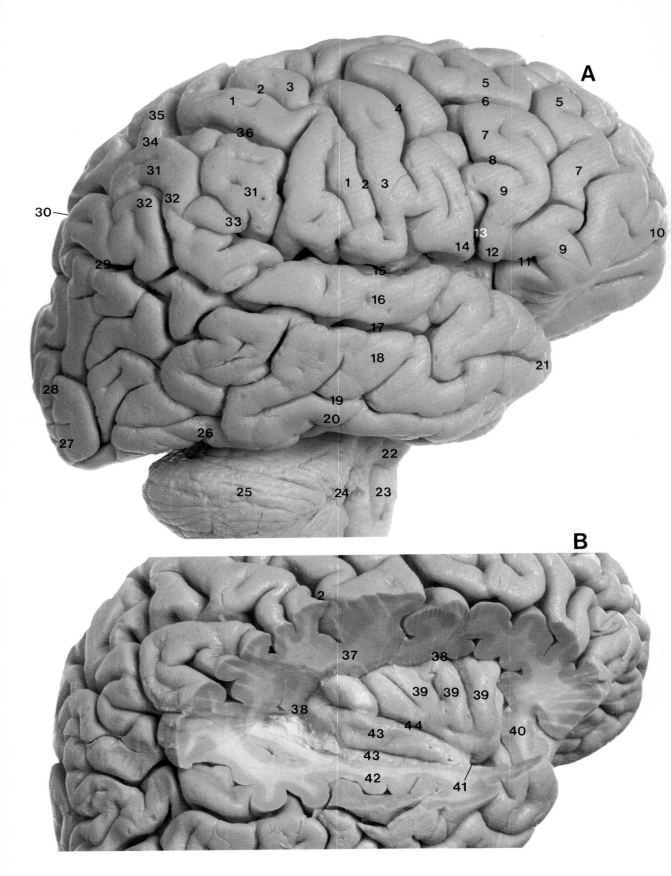

THE BRAIN

The cerebral hemisphere

A **The sulci and gyri of the superolateral surface of the right cerebral hemisphere**
B **The right insula after removal of its overlying opercula**

1 Postcentral gyrus
2 Central sulcus
3 Precentral gyrus
4 Precentral sulcus
5 Superior frontal gyrus
6 Superior frontal sulcus
7 Middle frontal gyrus
8 Inferior frontal sulcus
9 Inferior frontal gyrus
10 Frontal pole
11 Anterior ramus of lateral sulcus
12 Pars triangularis of inferior frontal gyrus
13 Ascending ramus of lateral sulcus
14 Pars opercularis of inferior frontal gyrus
15 Lateral sulcus (posterior ramus)
16 Superior temporal gyrus
17 Superior temporal sulcus
18 Middle temporal gyrus
19 Inferior temporal sulcus
20 Inferior temporal gyrus
21 Temporal pole
22 Pons
23 Medulla oblongata
24 Flocculus
25 Cerebellar hemisphere
26 Pre-occipital notch
27 Occipital pole
28 Lunate sulcus
29 Transverse occipital sulcus
30 Parieto-occipital sulcus
31 Inferior parietal lobule
32 Angular gyrus
33 Supramarginal gyrus
34 Intraparietal sulcus
35 Superior parietal lobule
36 Postcentral sulcus
37 Frontoparietal operculum
38 Circular sulcus of insula
39 Short gyri of insula
40 Frontal operculum
41 Limen of insula
42 Temporal operculum
43 Long gyri of insula
44 Central sulcus of insula

● The cerebral hemisphere has frontal, parietal, occipital and temporal lobes.

● The frontal lobe is the part lying in front of the central sulcus.

● The parietal lobe is bounded in front by the central sulcus and behind by the upper part of a line drawn from the parieto-occipital sulcus to the pre-occipital notch. The lower limit is the posterior ramus of the lateral sulcus (and an arbitrary line continued backwards in the main line of this ramus to the posterior boundary.

● The occipital lobe lies behind the line joining the parieto-occipital sulcus to the pre-occipital notch.

● The temporal lobe lies below the lateral sulcus, and is bounded behind by the lower part of the line drawn from the parieto-occipital sulcus to the pre-occipital notch.

● The lateral sulcus consists of short anterior and ascending rami, and a longer posterior ramus which itself is commonly known as the lateral sulcus.
● The areas around the anterior and ascending rami of the lateral sulcus of the left cerebral hemisphere constitute the motor speech area (of Broca).

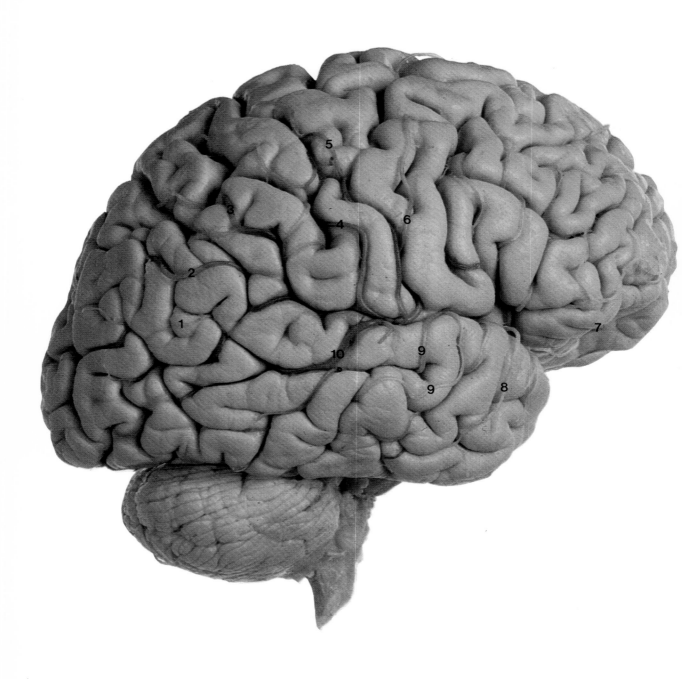

THE BRAIN

The middle cerebral artery on the lateral surface of the cerebral hemisphere

1 Artery of angular gyrus	⎫	
2 Posterior parietal artery		branches of
3 Anterior parietal artery		terminal
4 Artery of postcentral sulcus	⎬	(cortical) part
5 Artery of central sulcus		
6 Artery of precentral sulcus	⎭	
7 Lateral frontobasal artery		
8 Anterior temporal artery	⎫	branches of
9 Intermediate temporal artery	⎬	insular part
10 Posterior temporal artery	⎭	

● The middle cerebral artery supplies a large part of the lateral aspect of the cerebral cortex, except for a strip along the upper border (anterior cerebral) and lower border (posterior cerebral). The cortex supplied includes much of the motor area of the precentral gyrus (but excluding the 'leg area', supplied by the anterior cerebral), the auditory area of the superior temporal gyrus, and the insula (in the depths of the lateral sulcus). Some small middle cerebral branches extend as far back as the most lateral part of the visual area of the cortex (see page 183).

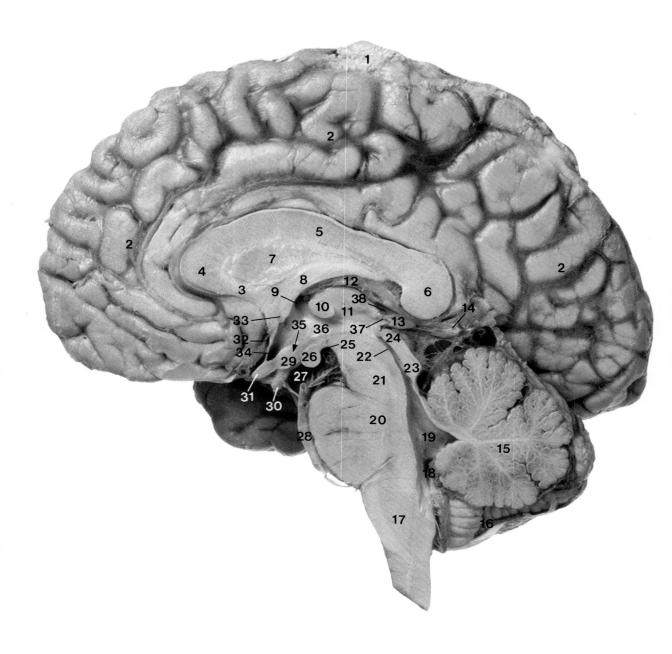

THE BRAIN

A median sagittal section

The right half, from the left *(with the arachnoid mater and blood vessels intact)*

1 Arachnoid granulations
2 Arachnoid mater and vessels overlying medial surface of cerebral hemisphere
3 Rostrum ⎫
4 Genu ⎪
5 Body ⎬ of corpus callosum
6 Splenium ⎭
7 Septum pellucidum
8 Body of fornix
9 Interventricular foramen
10 Interthalamic adhesion
11 Third ventricle
12 Choroid plexus of third ventricle
13 Pineal body
14 Great cerebral vein
15 Cerebellum
16 Cerebellomedullary cistern (cisterna magna)
17 Medulla oblongata
18 Choroid plexus of fourth ventricle
19 Fourth ventricle
20 Pons
21 Midbrain
22 Aqueduct of midbrain
23 Inferior colliculus
24 Superior colliculus
25 Posterior perforated substance
26 Mamillary body
27 Interpeduncular cistern
28 Basilar artery
29 Tuber cinereum
30 Pituitary stalk
31 Optic chiasma
32 Lamina terminalis
33 Anterior commissure
34 Optic recess
35 Infundibular recess
36 Hypothalamus
37 Pineal recess
38 Suprapineal recess

● The midbrain consists of the two cerebral peduncles.
● Each cerebral peduncle consists of a ventral part, the crus of the peduncle and a dorsal part, the tegmentum with an intervening layer of pigmented grey matter, the substantia nigra.
● The tegmentum contains the aqueduct of the midbrain; the part of the tegmentum dorsal to the aqueduct is the tectum, and includes the superior and inferior colliculi.

● The pituitary gland is properly known as the hypophysis cerebri, and can be divided into two regions, the adenohypophysis and neurohypophysis.
● The adenohypophysis is derived from an outgrowth of ectoderm from the primitive mouth (Rathke's pouch) and consists of the pars distalis (pars anterior), pars tuberalis and pars intermedia.
● The neurohypophysis is derived from an outgrowth of neurectoderm from the primitive forebrain and consists of the pars nervosa, infundibulum and median eminence.
● The term 'anterior lobe of the pituitary' is commonly understood to be equivalent to the pars distalis (pars anterior), and 'posterior lobe of the pituitary' to mean the pars nervosa.
● The infundibulum, or infundibular part, of the pituitary stalk is the upper hollow part containing the infundibular recess of the third ventricle.
● The tuber cinereum, between the mamillary bodies and the optic chiasma, includes an area at the base of the infundibulum known as the median eminence, which is important as a site of neurosecretory cells whose products enter the hypophysial portal system of blood vessels to control the hormones of the adenohypophysis.

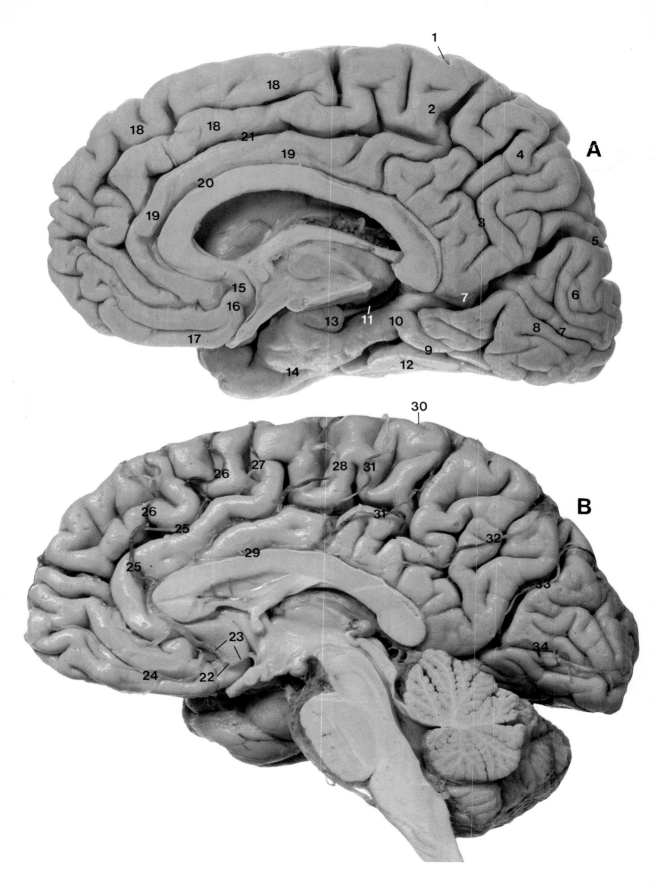

THE BRAIN

The medial surface of the cerebral hemisphere and the anterior and posterior cerebral arteries

A The sulci and gyri of the medial surface of the right cerebral hemisphere, with the brainstem removed

1 Central sulcus
2 Paracentral lobule
3 Subparietal sulcus
4 Precuneus
5 Parieto-occipital sulcus
6 Cuneus
7 Calcarine sulcus
8 Lingual gyrus
9 Collateral sulcus
10 Parahippocampal gyrus
11 Dentate gyrus
12 Medial occipitotemporal gyrus
13 Uncus
14 Rhinal sulcus
15 Paraterminal gyrus
16 Subcallosal area
17 Gyrus rectus
18 Medial frontal gyrus
19 Cingulate gyrus
20 Corpus callosal sulcus
21 Cingulate sulcus

B The anterior and posterior cerebral arteries on the medial surface of the right cerebral hemisphere

22 Anterior communicating artery
23 Anterior cerebral artery
24 Medial frontobasal artery
25 Callosomarginal artery
26 Anteromedial frontal arteries
27 Intermediomedial frontal artery   } from the
28 Posteromedial frontal artery   anterior
29 Pericallosal artery   cerebral
30 Central sulcus   artery
31 Paracentral artery
32 Precuneal artery
33 Parieto-occipital branch } of posterior
34 Calcarine branch   } cerebral artery

● On the surface of the cerebral hemisphere the anterior cerebral artery supplies the cortex on the medial aspect as far back as the parieto-occipital sulcus, and a strip on the upper part of the lateral surface adjacent to the midline (i.e. the supply 'spills over' from the medial surface of the hemisphere on to the superolateral surface). The cortex supplied includes the 'leg area' of the motor cortex.

● The posterior cerebral artery supplies the cortex of the occipital lobe and an area continuing forwards on the medial and inferior surfaces of the temporal lobe as far as and including the uncus (but not including the temporal pole which has a middle cerebral supply). The cortex supplied includes the visual area (striate cortex) which is found principally in the upper and lower lips of the posterior part of the calcarine sulcus and extending as far as the lunate sulcus in the region of the occipital pole. Here there is some anastomosis with branches from the middle cerebral artery which results in the 'macular area' of the visual cortex receiving a middle cerebral supply.

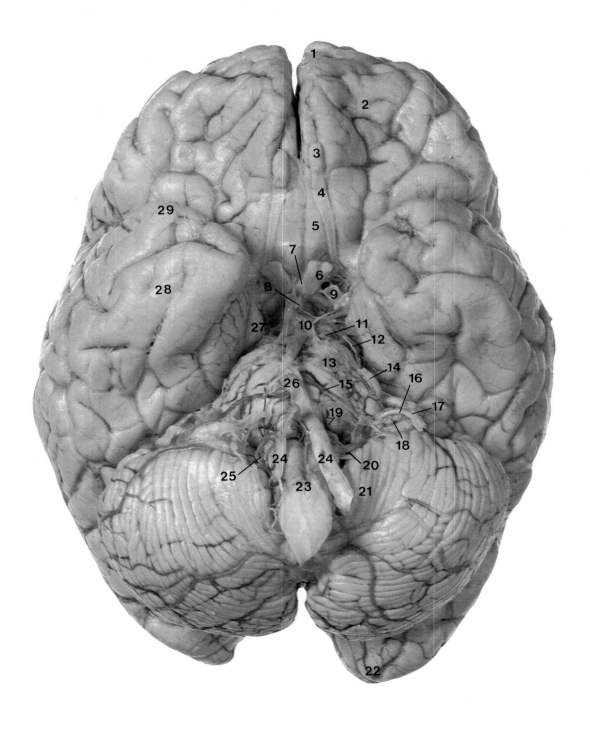

THE BRAIN

The base of the brain

From below *(with some adherent arachnoid mater, as typically seen after removal from the cranial cavity and before any dissection)*

1 Frontal pole
2 Inferior surface of frontal lobe
3 Olfactory bulb
4 Olfactory tract
5 Gyrus rectus
6 Optic nerve
7 Optic chiasma
8 Pituitary stalk
9 Internal carotid artery
10 Arachnoid mater overlying mamillary bodies
11 Oculomotor nerve
12 Trochlear nerve
13 Pons
14 Trigeminal nerve
15 Labyrinthine artery
16 Facial nerve
17 Vestibulocochlear nerve
18 Flocculus
19 Abducent nerve
20 Rootlets of glossopharyngeal, vagus and cranial part of accessory nerves
21 Tonsil of cerebellum
22 Occipital pole
23 Medulla oblongata
24 Vertebral artery
25 Posterior inferior cerebellar artery
26 Basilar artery
27 Uncus
28 Inferior surface of temporal lobe
29 Temporal pole

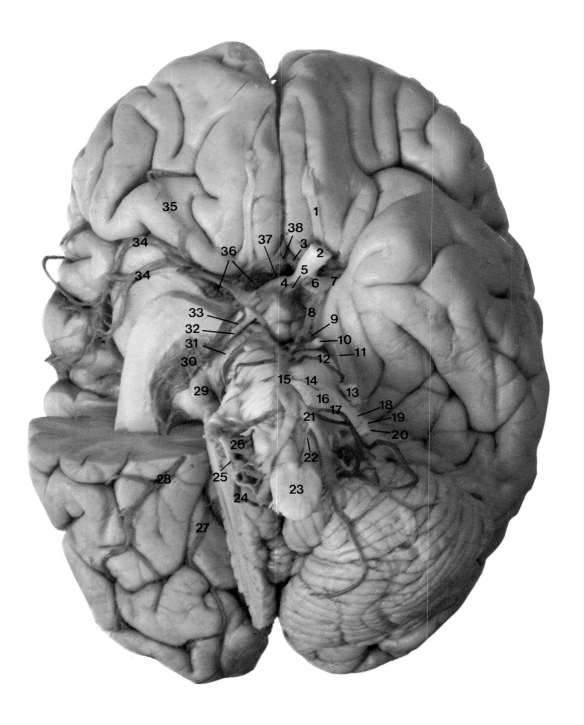

THE BRAIN

The base of the brain and the arterial circle

From below *(after removal of part of the right temporal lobe and cerebellar hemisphere)*

1 Olfactory tract
2 Optic nerve
3 Anterior cerebral artery
4 Optic chiasma
5 Pituitary stalk
6 Internal carotid artery
7 Middle cerebral artery
8 Posterior communicating artery
9 Posterior cerebral artery
10 Oculomotor nerve
11 Trochlear nerve
12 Superior cerebellar artery
13 Trigeminal nerve
14 Labyrinthine artery
15 Basilar artery
16 Pons
17 Anterior inferior cerebellar artery
18 Middle cerebellar peduncle
19 Facial nerve
20 Vestibulocochlear nerve
21 Vertebral artery
22 Anterior spinal artery
23 Medulla oblongata
24 Posterior inferior cerebellar artery
25 Spinal root of accessory nerve
26 Rootlets of glossopharyngeal, vagus and cranial part of accessory nerves
27 Posterior temporal ⎫ branches of posterior
28 Middle temporal ⎭ cerebral artery
29 Lateral geniculate body
30 Choroid plexus of inferior horn of lateral ventricle
31 Cerebral peduncle
32 Optic tract
33 Anterior choroidal artery
34 Cortical branches of middle cerebral artery
35 Lateral frontobasal artery
36 Striate branches of middle and anterior cerebral arteries
37 Long central (recurrent) branch of anterior cerebral artery
38 Anterior communicating artery

● The arterial circle (of Willis) is an anastomosis (hexagonal rather than circular in shape) between the internal carotid and vertebral systems of vessels. The anterior cerebral branches of each internal carotid artery are joined by the (single) anterior communicating artery; on each side a posterior communicating artery joins the internal carotid to the posterior cerebral artery, the two posterior cerebrals being the terminal branches of the (midline) basilar artery (which has been formed by the union of the two vertebrals).

● The various striate branches of the middle and anterior cerebral arteries which enter the anterior perforated substance supply (among other structures) the internal capsule. One such branch of the middle cerebral artery has become known as the 'artery of cerebral haemorrhage' since it is particularly liable to rupture and thus damage corticonuclear and corticospinal fibres that course through the posterior limb of the capsule. This type of cerebral damage which causes varying degrees of paralysis, especially of the limbs, is popularly known as a 'stroke'.

A

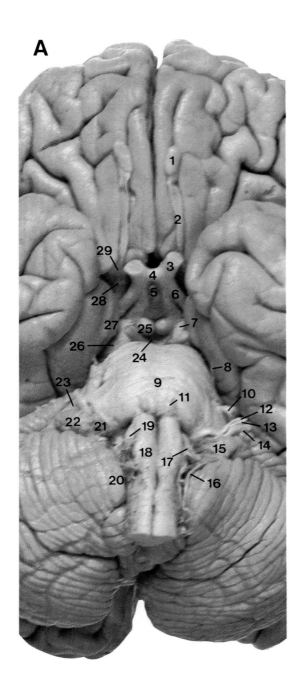

B

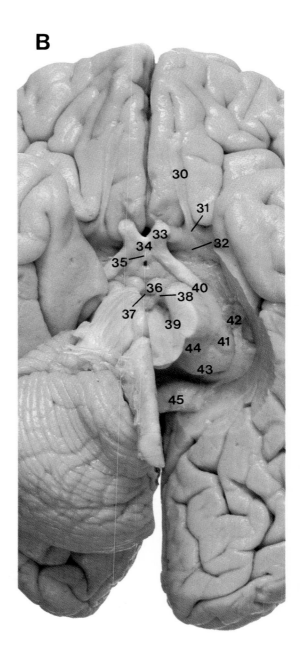

THE BRAIN

The brainstem, cranial nerves and geniculate bodies

A The brainstem and cranial nerves, from below *(after removal of the meninges and blood vessels)*

1 Olfactory bulb
2 Olfactory tract
3 Optic nerve
4 Optic chiasma
5 Pituitary stalk
6 Optic tract
7 Oculomotor nerve
8 Trochlear nerve
9 Pons
10 Trigeminal nerve
11 Abducent nerve
12 Motor⎫
13 Sensory root⎭ of facial nerve
14 Vestibulocochlear nerve
15 Roots of glossopharyngeal, vagus and cranial part of accessory nerves
16 Spinal root of accessory nerve
17 Rootlets of hypoglossal nerve
18 Pyramid of medulla oblongata
19 Olive
20 Tonsil of cerebellum
21 Choroid plexus of fourth ventricle
22 Flocculus
23 Middle cerebellar peduncle
24 Posterior perforated substance
25 Mamillary body
26 Cerebral peduncle
27 Uncus
28 Anterior perforated substance
29 Olfactory trigone

B The left optic tract and geniculate bodies, from below *(after removal of part of the brainstem, cerebellum and cerebral hemisphere)*

30 Olfactory tract
31 Olfactory trigone
32 Anterior perforated substance
33 Optic nerve
34 Optic chiasma
35 Pituitary stalk
36 Mamillary body
37 Posterior perforated substance
38 Oculomotor nerve
39 Cerebral peduncle
40 Optic tract
41 Lateral geniculate body
42 Choroid plexus of inferior horn of lateral ventricle
43 Pulvinar
44 Medial geniculate body
45 Splenium of corpus callosum

● The cranial nerves are numbered as well as named:

First	olfactory
Second	optic
Third	oculomotor
Fourth	trochlear
Fifth	trigeminal
Sixth	abducent
Seventh	facial
Eighth	vestibulocochlear
Ninth	glossopharyngeal
Tenth	vagus
Eleventh	accessory
Twelfth	hypoglossal

● The olfactory nerve consists of about 20 filaments that pass through the cribriform plate of the ethmoid bone.

● The optic nerve passes backwards from the eye through the optic canal to the optic chiasma.

● The trochlear nerve is the only cranial nerve to emerge from the *dorsal* surface of the brainstem (from the midbrain, behind the inferior colliculus).

● The oculomotor nerve *emerges* on the *medial* side of the cerebral penduncle, and the trochlear nerve winds round the *lateral* side of the peduncle. Both nerves pass between the posterior cerebral and superior cerebellar arteries.

● The trigeminal nerve emerges from the lateral side of the pons, where the pons continues into the middle cerebellar peduncle.

● The abducent nerve emerges between the pons and the pyramid.

● The facial and vestibulocochlear nerves emerge from the lateral pontomedullary angle.

● The glossopharyngeal and vagus nerves and the cranial part of the accessory nerve emerge from the medulla oblongata lateral to the olive.

● The spinal part of the accessory nerve emerges as a series of roots from the lateral surface of the upper five or six segments of the spinal cord, dorsal to the denticulate ligament.

● The hypoglossal nerve emerges between the pyramid and the olive.

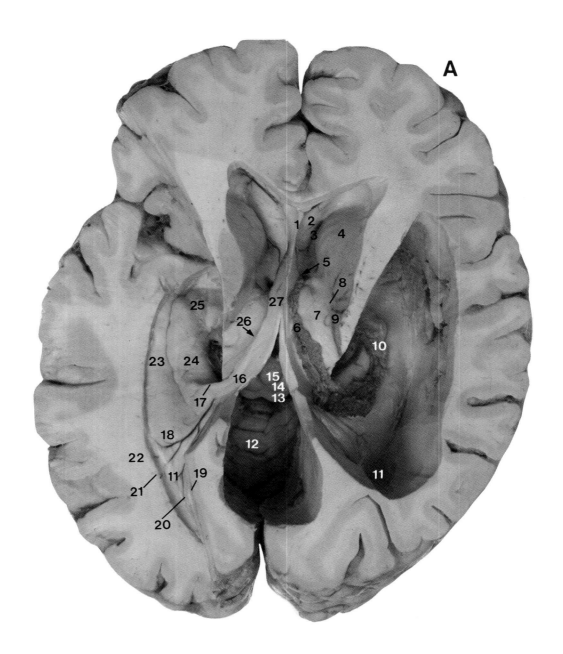

A

THE BRAIN

The third ventricle and the lateral ventricles

A The lateral ventricles and their horns, dissected
from above
B The roof of the third ventricle, from above

1 Septum pellucidum
2 Rostrum of corpus callosum (posterior surface)
3 Anterior horn of lateral ventricle
4 Head of caudate nucleus
5 Interventricular foramen
6 Choroid plexus of body of lateral ventricle

7 Thalamus
8 Thalamostriate vein
9 Body of caudate nucleus
10 Choroid plexus of inferior horn of lateral
ventricle
11 Posterior horn of lateral ventricle
12 Vermis of cerebellum
13 Inferior colliculus
14 Superior colliculus
15 Pineal body
16 Crus of fornix
17 Fimbria
18 Collateral trigone
19 Bulb
20 Calcar
21 Tapetum of corpus callosum
22 Optic radiation
23 Collateral eminence
24 Hippocampus
25 Pes hippocampi
26 Choroid fissure
27 Body of fornix
28 Anterior column of fornix
29 Tela choroidea of third ventricle
30 Choroid plexus in third ventricle (visible below
29)
31 Internal cerebral vein
32 Great cerebral vein

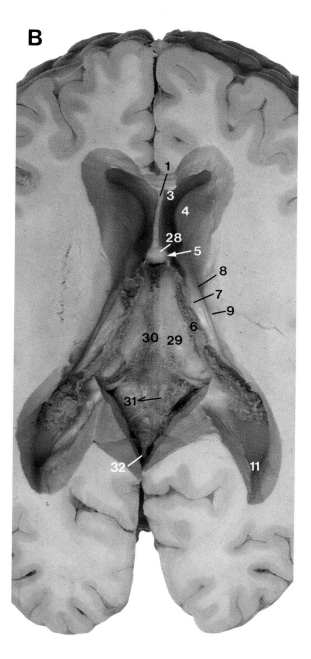

● The ventricles of the brain:
the third ventricle, with on each side an interventricular
foramen *leading into*
the lateral ventricle, consisting of a body with anterior,
posterior and inferior horns
the aqueduct of the midbrain, connecting the third ventricle
with
the fourth ventricle, which has a median aperture (in the
roof) and a lateral aperture (in each lateral recess)
through which cerebrospinal fluid escapes into the
subarachnoid space.

● Tela choroidea is the name given to a double layer of pia
mater. When it contains a mass of capillary blood vessels and is
covered by ependyma (the epithelium lining the ventricles) it
becomes the choroid plexus.

● Cerebrospinal fluid is produced by the choroid plexus
which is in the roof of the third ventricle and extends through
each interventricular foramen into the body and then the
inferior horn of the lateral ventricle (but *not* into the anterior
or posterior horns). A separate choroid plexus, not connected
with the above, lies in the roof of the fourth ventricle and
extends out through the lateral recesses.

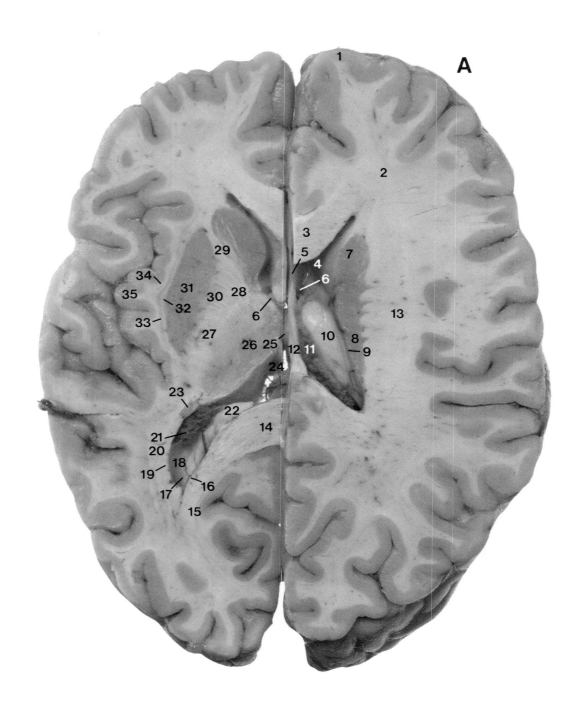

A

THE BRAIN

The internal capsule and basal nuclei in horizontal sections of the cerebral hemispheres

A From above (*the left hemisphere sectioned through the interventricular foramen, and the right hemisphere 1 cm higher*)

B The left hemisphere, from below (*at a slightly lower level than the left side in A*)

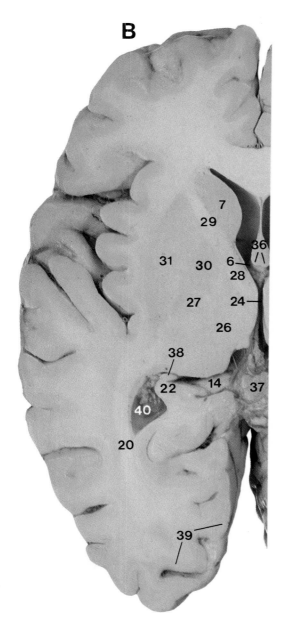

1 Frontal pole
2 Forceps minor
3 Genu of corpus callosum
4 Anterior horn of lateral ventricle
5 Septum pellucidum
6 Interventricular foramen
7 Head ⎫
8 Body ⎬ of caudate nucleus
9 Thalomostriate vein
10 Thalamus
11 Choroid plexus of body of lateral ventricle
12 Body of fornix
13 Corona radiata
14 Splenium of corpus callosum
15 Forceps major
16 Bulb
17 Calcar
18 Posterior horn of lateral ventricle
19 Tapetum of corpus callosum
20 Optic radiation
21 Choroid plexus passing forwards into inferior horn of lateral ventricle
22 Crus of fornix
23 Tail of caudate nucleus
24 Third ventricle
25 Interthalamic adhesion
26 Thalamus
27 Posterior limb ⎫
28 Genu ⎬ of internal capsule
29 Anterior limb ⎭
30 Globus pallidus ⎫
31 Putamen ⎬ lentiform nucleus
32 External capsule
33 Claustrum
34 Extreme capsule
35 Insula
36 Anterior column of fornix
37 Pineal body
38 Fimbria
39 Visual (striate) area of cerebral cortex
40 Junction of posterior and inferior horns of lateral ventricle

● Among the most important of the fibres that pass through the internal capsule, mainly through its posterior limb, are corticonuclear fibres (formerly called corticobulbar) to the motor nuclei of cranial nerves, and corticospinal fibres to anterior horn cells of the spinal cord.

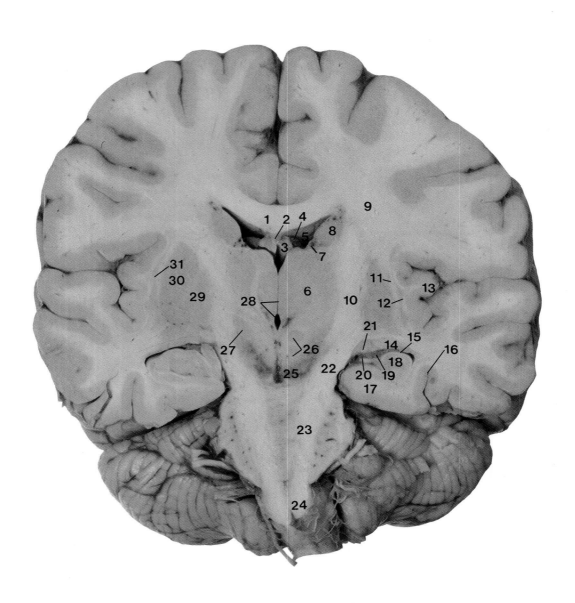

THE BRAIN

The cerebral hemispheres and brainstem in coronal section

From the front *(slightly oblique, on a plane from behind the interventricular foramen and through the pyramids of the medulla oblongata)*

 1 Corpus callosum
 2 Septum pellucidum
 3 Body of fornix
 4 Choroid plexus
 5 Body of lateral ventricle
 6 Thalamus
 7 Thalamostriate vein
 8 Body of caudate nucleus
 9 Corona radiata
10 Internal capsule
11 External capsule
12 Extreme capsule
13 Insula
14 Tail of caudate nucleus
15 Inferior horn of lateral ventricle
16 Collateral sulcus
17 Parahippocampal gyrus
18 Hippocampus
19 Choroid plexus of inferior horn of lateral ventricle
20 Choroid fissure
21 Optic tract
22 Corticospinal and corticonuclear fibres in cerebral peduncle
23 Corticospinal and corticonuclear fibres in pons
24 Corticospinal fibres in pyramid of medulla oblongata
25 Substantia nigra
26 Red nucleus
27 Subthalamic nucleus
28 Third ventricle
29 Globus pallidus ⎫ lentiform nucleus
30 Putamen   ⎭
31 Claustrum

● Groups of nerve cells *within* the central nervous system are usually called nuclei.

● Groups of nerve cells *outside* the central nervous system i.e. in the peripheral nervous system associated with the afferent fibres of cranial and spinal nerves and with autonomic nerves, are called ganglia.

● The myelinated fibres from nerve cells of the cerebral cortex pass through the white matter of the cerebral hemisphere and can be classified into three groups according to their courses and connexions:
   Association (arcuate) fibres, passing from one area of cerebral cortex to another part of the cortex of the same hemisphere
   Commissural fibres, passing from one cerebral hemisphere to the corresponding area of the opposite hemisphere
   Projection fibres, passing from the cerebral cortex to the grey matter of the brainstem and spinal cord (and including fibres passing in the opposite direction)

● The basal nuclei (formerly known as the basal ganglia) consist of:
   the caudate nucleus
   the lentiform nucleus
   the amygdaloid nucleus
   the claustrum
● The lentiform nucleus consists of the putamen and globus pollidus.
● The corpus striatum consists of the caudate and lentiform nuclei.

● The thalamus is a large group of cells in its own right, subdivided into a number of nuclei, and should not be included among the basal nuclei.

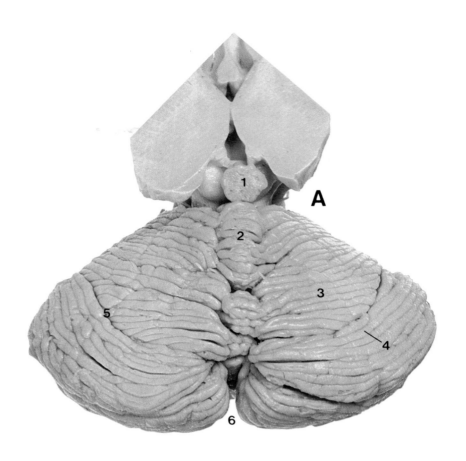

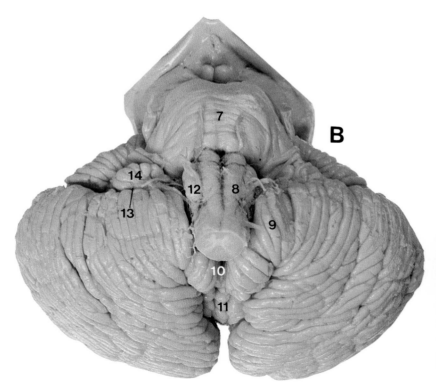

THE BRAIN

The cerebellum and brainstem

A From above
B From below

1 Pineal body
2 Vermis of cerebellum
3 Cerebellar hemisphere
4 A cerebellar folium
5 Primary fissure
6 Cerebellar notch
7 Pons
8 Pyramid of medulla oblongata
9 Tonsil of cerebellum
10 Uvula of vermis
11 Pyramid of vermis
12 Olive
13 Dorsolateral (posterolateral) fissure
14 Flocculus

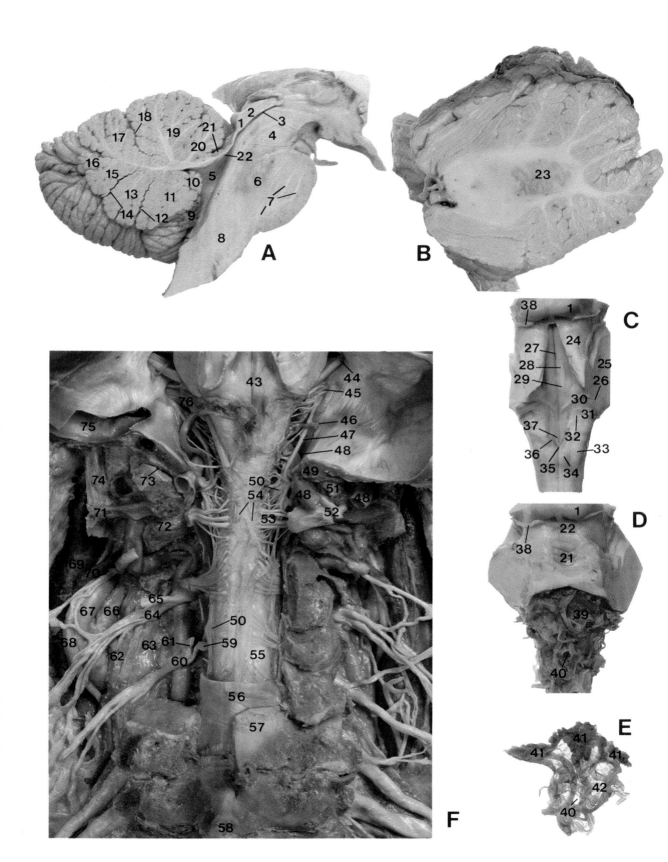

198

The Brain and Spinal Cord

The cerebellum, brainstem and fourth ventricle, and the spinal cord

A **The left half of a midline sagittal section**
B **An oblique sagittal section through the left cerebellar hemisphere, from the left**
C **The floor of the fourth ventricle** *(the brainstem from behind, with the cerebellum removed)*
D **The roof of the fourth ventricle** *(the brainstem from behind, with most of the cerebellum removed)*
E **The isolated choroid plexus of the fourth ventricle**

 1 Inferior colliculus
 2 Tectum ⎫
 3 Aqueduct ⎬ of midbrain
 4 Tegmentum ⎭
 5 Fourth ventricle
 6 Pons
 7 Corticonuclear and corticospinal fibres
 8 Medulla oblongata
 9 Choroid plexus of fourth ventricle
10 Nodule
11 Uvula of vermis
12 Secondary (postpyramidal) fissure
13 Pyramid of vermis
14 Prepyramidal fissure
15 Tuber of vermis
16 Folium of vermis
17 Declive
18 Primary fissure
19 Culmen
20 Central lobule
21 Lingula
22 Superior medullary velum
23 Dentate nucleus
24 Superior ⎫
25 Middle ⎬ cerebellar peduncle
26 Inferior ⎭
27 Median groove
28 Medial eminence
29 Facial colliculus
30 Medullary striae
31 Lateral recess
32 Vestibular area
33 Cuneate tubercle
34 Gracile tubercle
35 Obex
36 Vagal triangle
37 Hypoglossal triangle
38 Trochlear nerve
39 Tela choroidea and choroid plexus
40 Median aperture
41 Choroid plexus
42 Tela choroidea

F **The lower brainstem and cervical part of the spinal cord, from behind** *(after removal of the cerebellum and parts of the skull and cervical vertebrae)*

43 Floor of fourth ventricle
44 Internal acoustic meatus with facial and vestibulocochlear nerves and labyrinthine artery
45 Roots of glossopharyngeal, vagus and cranial part of accessory nerves
46 Posterior inferior cerebellar artery
47 Spinal root of accessory nerve
48 Vertebral artery
49 Margin of foramen magnum
50 Denticulate ligament
51 Lateral mass of atlas
52 First cervical nerve and posterior arch of atlas
53 Dorsal rootlets of second cervical nerve
54 Posterior spinal arteries
55 Arachnoid mater
56 Dura mater
57 Lamina of sixth cervical vertebra
58 Spinous process of seventh cervical vertebra
59 Ventral rootlets ⎫
60 Dorsal root ganglion ⎬ of fourth cervical nerve
61 Dorsal root ⎭
62 Scalenus anterior
63 Longus capitis
64 Ventral ramus ⎫ of third cervical nerve
65 Dorsal ramus ⎭
66 External carotid artery
67 Internal carotid artery
68 Vagus nerve
69 Internal jugular vein
70 A vein from vertebral venous plexuses
71 Transverse process of atlas
72 Capsule of lateral atlanto-axial joint
73 Atlanto-occipital joint
74 Rectus capitis lateralis
75 Sigmoid sinus
76 Choroid plexus emerging from lateral recess of fourth ventricle

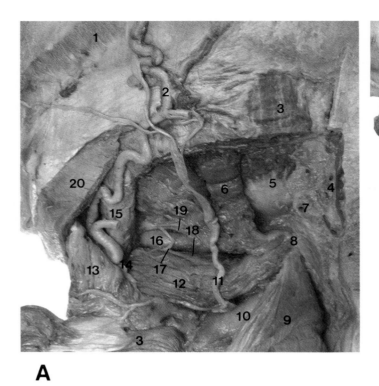

A

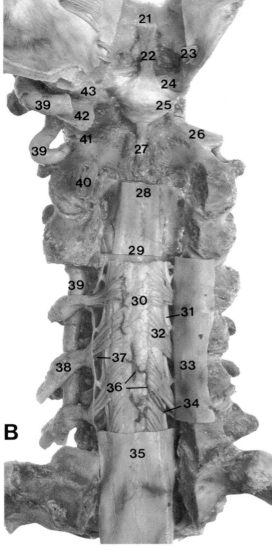

B

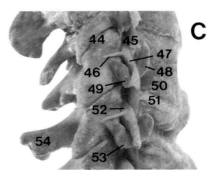

C

THE BRAIN AND SPINAL CORD

The suboccipital triangle, vertebral column and spinal cord and intervertebral foramina
(For the vertebral column from the front see page 108)

A The left suboccipital triangle *(exposed after removing or reflecting trapezius, splenius capitis and semispinalis capitis)*

1 Occipital belly of occipitofrontalis
2 Occipital artery
3 Semispinalis capitis
4 Ligamentum nuchae
5 Rectus capitis posterior minor
6 Rectus capitis posterior major
7 Posterior tubercle of atlas
8 Spinous process of axis
9 Semispinalis cervicis
10 Lamina of axis
11 Greater occipital nerve
12 Obliquus capitis inferior
13 Longissimus capitis
14 Transverse process of atlas
15 Obliquus capitis superior
16 Vertebral artery
17 Dorsal ramus of first cervical nerve
18 Posterior arch of atlas
19 Posterior atlanto-occipital membrane
20 Splenius capitis

B The vertebral column and spinal cord, from behind *(after removal of the vertebral arches)*

21 Basilar part of occipital bone and position of attachment of tectorial membrane
22 Superior longitudinal band of cruciform ligament
23 Hypoglossal nerve and canal
24 Alar ligament
25 Transverse ligament of atlas
26 Superior articular surface of axis
27 Inferior longitudinal band of cruciform ligament
28 Tectorial membrane
29 Posterior longitudinal ligament
30 Spinal cord
31 Denticulate ligament
32 Dorsal rootlets of spinal nerve
33 Arachnoid and dura mater (reflected)
34 Radicular artery
35 Dura mater
36 Posterior spinal arteries
37 Ventral rootlets of spinal nerve
38 Dural sheath over dorsal root ganglion
39 Vertebral artery
40 Pedicle of axis
41 Lateral atlanto-axial joint
42 Posterior arch of atlas
43 Atlanto-occipital joint

C Intervertebral foramina and the rami of spinal nerves, from the right *(in part of the cervical vertebral column)*

44 Zygapophysial joint
45 Vertebral artery
46 Dorsal ramus } of fourth cervical nerve
47 Ventral ramus
48 Anterior tubercle } of transverse process
49 Posterior tubercle
50 Body of fourth cervical vertebra
51 Intervertebral disc
52 Dorsal root ganglion of fifth cervical nerve in intervertebral foramen
53 Groove for (ventral ramus of) spinal nerve
54 Spinous process of fifth cervical vertebra

● Suboccipital triangle
   Boundaries: rectus capitis posterior major, obliquus capitis superior and obliquus capitis inferior.
   Floor: posterior atlanto-occipital membrane and posterior arch of the atlas.
   Contents: vertebral artery and the dorsal ramus of the first cervical nerve.

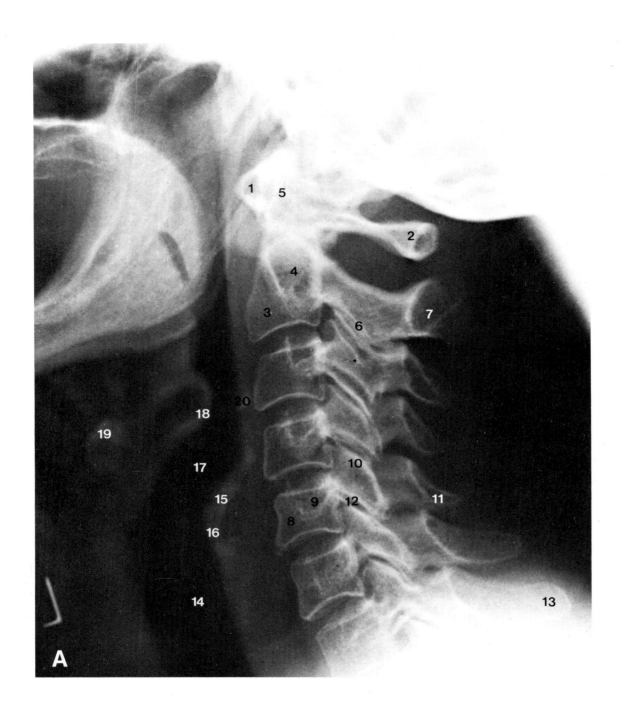

Radiographs of Head and Neck

Cervical vertebral column

A Lateral view
B Anteroposterior view
C Oblique view

1 Anterior arch } of atlas
2 Posterior arch
3 Body
4 Transverse process
5 Dens } of axis
6 Inferior articular process
7 Spinous process

8 Body
9 Transverse process } of fifth cervical vertebra
10 Superior articular process
11 Spinous process
12 Zygapophysial joint
13 Spinous process of seventh cervical vertebra
14 Trachea
15 Calcification in arytenoid cartilage
16 Calcification in thyroid cartilage
17 Vestibule of larynx
18 Epiglottis
19 Body } of hyoid bone
20 Tip of greater horn
21 Lateral mass } of atlas
22 Transverse process
23 Lateral atlanto-axial joint
24 Uncus of body of fifth cervical vertebra
25 Body } of fourth cervical vertebra
26 Pedicle
27 Intervertebral foramen
28 Pedicle of fifth cervical vertebra
29 Intervertebral disc

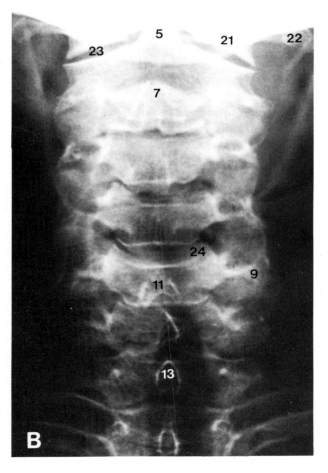

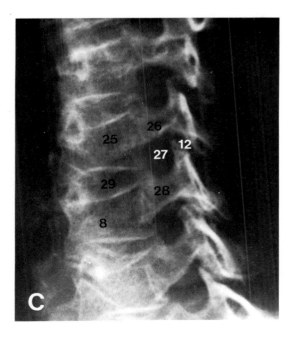

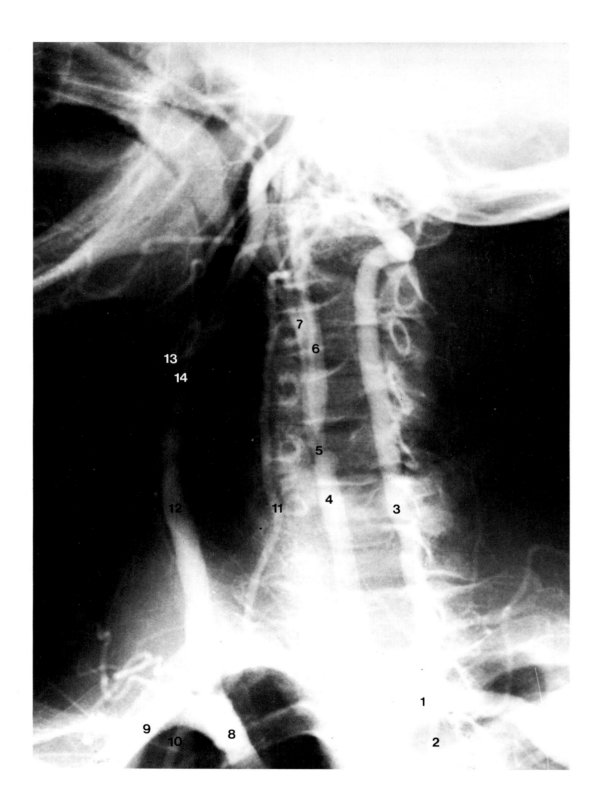

RADIOGRAPHS OF HEAD AND NECK

The upper part of an arch aortogram, oblique view, showing vessels in the neck *(The left vertebral artery is abnormally large due to back pressure from a pathological constriction in the left common carotid artery)*

 1 Left subclavian artery
 2 Left internal thoracic artery
 3 Left vertebral artery (abnormally large)
 4 Left common carotid artery
 5 Constriction in **4**
 6 Left internal carotid artery
 7 Left external carotid artery
 8 Brachiocephalic artery
 9 Right subclavian artery
10 Right internal thoracic artery
11 Right vertebral artery
12 Right common carotid artery
13 Right external carotid artery
14 Right internal carotid artery

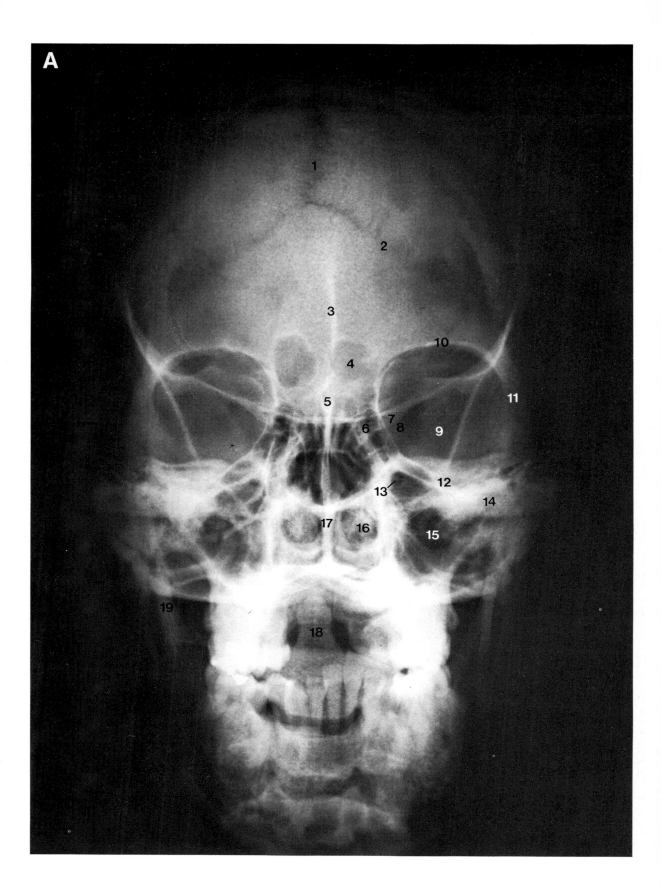

RADIOGRAPHS OF HEAD AND NECK

The head

A Postero-anterior view
B Occipitomental view *(for the paranasal sinuses)*

 1 Sagittal suture
 2 Lambdoid suture
 3 Calcification in falx cerebri
 4 Frontal sinus
 5 Crista galli
 6 Ethmoidal air cells
 7 Lesser wing of sphenoid bone
 8 Superior orbital fissure
 9 Greater wing of sphenoid bone
10 Supra-orbital margin
11 Frontozygomatic suture
12 Infra-orbital margin
13 Foramen rotundum
14 Petrous part of temporal bone
15 Maxillary sinus
16 Inferior nasal concha
17 Nasal septum
18 Dens of axis
19 Coronoid process of mandible
20 Zygomatic bone
21 Zygomatic arch

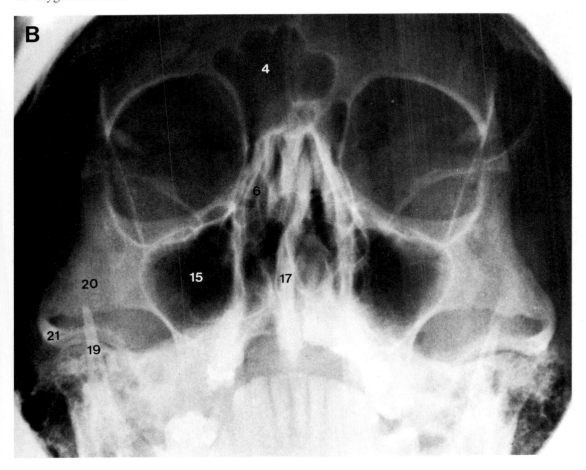

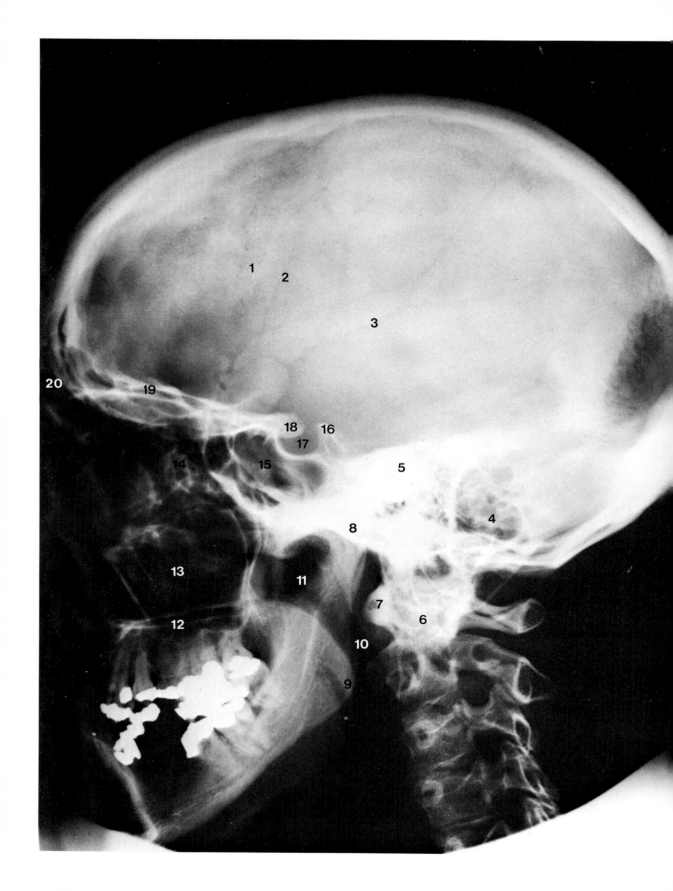

RADIOGRAPHS OF HEAD AND NECK

The head

Lateral view

1 Coronal suture
2 Frontal branch ⎫ of middle meningeal
3 Parietal branch ⎭ artery
4 Mastoid air cells
5 External acoustic meatus
6 Mastoid process
7 Anterior arch of atlas
8 Head ⎫ of mandible
9 Angle ⎭
10 Oral part ⎫ of pharynx
11 Nasal part ⎭
12 Hard palate
13 Maxillary sinus
14 Ethmoidal air cells
15 Sphenoidal sinus
16 Posterior clinoid process
17 Pituitary fossa
18 Anterior clinoid process
19 Floor of anterior cranial fossa
20 Frontal sinus

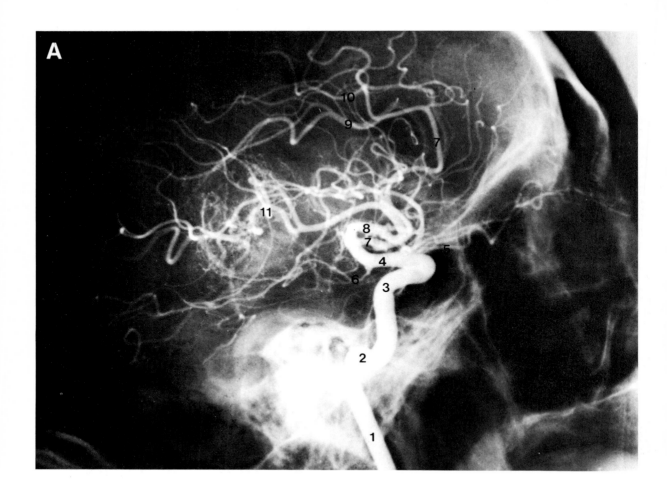

RADIOGRAPHS OF HEAD AND NECK

Carotid arteriograms

A Lateral view
B Anterior view

1 Cervical ⎫
2 Petrous ⎬ part of internal
3 Sphenoidal ⎥ carotid artery
4 Cerebral ⎭
5 Ophthalmic artery
6 Anterior choroidal artery
7 Anterior cerebral artery
8 Middle cerebral artery
9 Pericallosal artery
10 Callosomarginal artery
11 Branches of middle cerebral artery

● In arteriograms of the internal carotid artery, the curve of the vessel in and above the cavernous sinus (like the letter U on its side, as in A between 3 and 4) is commonly called the carotid siphon.

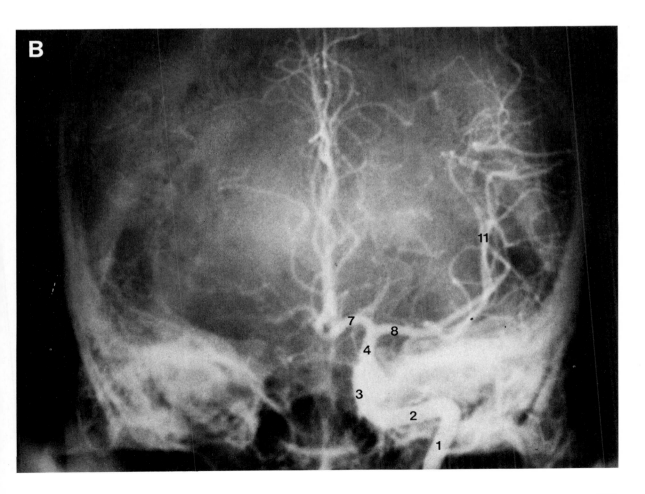

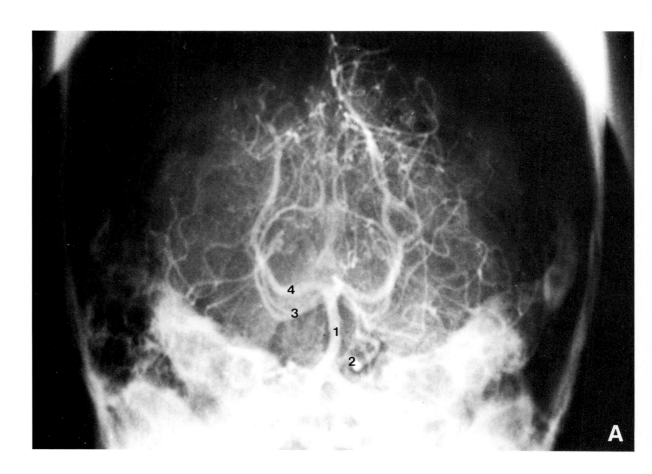

RADIOGRAPHS OF HEAD AND NECK

Vertebral arteriograms

A Anterior view
B Lateral view

(The vertebral arteries themselves are not clearly defined, but part of one can be identified in B)

1 Basilar artery
2 Anterior inferior cerebellar artery
3 Superior cerebellar artery
4 Posterior cerebral artery
5 Vertebral artery
6 Posterior choroidal arteries and choroid plexus of third ventricle

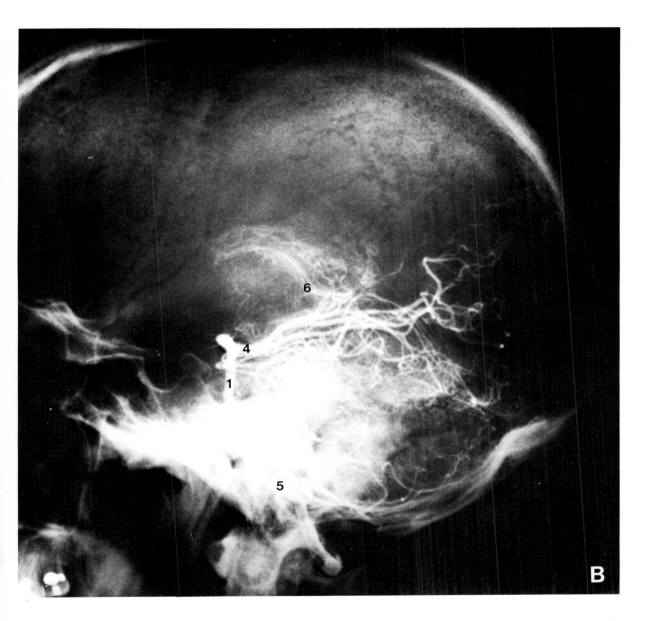

Appendix

The following lists are included to provide 'at-a-glance' reference to muscle groups, branches of nerves and arteries, tributaries of veins, and to lymph nodes. The nerves and vessels have been grouped to provide quick identification of parent trunks and branches, according to the indentation of the listed names. Thus the superior laryngeal artery is a branch of the superior thyroid, which in turn is a branch of the external carotid.

An arrow indicates a continuity with a change of name, not a branching.

The inclusion of items here does not necessarily imply that they are all illustrated in the atlas. Many of the smaller vessels and nerves in particular are not shown but have been included to provide a record of generally accepted terms as far as the anatomy of the head and neck is concerned.

A list of skull foramina with the structures that pass through them is also included but some students may find that the simplified list of the more important items on page 25 is sufficient for their purpose.

Muscles

MUSCLES OF THE HEAD
Muscles of the scalp
Epicranius
  Occipitofrontalis
    Occipital belly
    Frontal belly
  Temporoparietalis

Muscles of the auricle
Extrinsic
  Auricularis anterior
  Auricularis superior
  Auricularis posterior
Intrinsic
  Helicis major and minor
  Tragicus
  Antitragicus
  Transversus auriculae
  Obliquus auriculae

Muscles of the nose
Procerus
Nasalis
  Transverse part (compressor naris)
  Alar part (dilator naris)
Depressor septi

Muscles of the eyelids
Orbicularis oculi
  Orbital part
    Depressor supercilii
  Palpebral part
  Lacrimal part
Corrugator supercilii
Levator palpebrae superioris (see Muscles of the orbit)

Muscles of mastication
Temporalis
Masseter
Lateral pterygoid
Medial pterygoid

Muscles of the mouth
Levator labii superioris
Levator labii superioris alaeque nasi
Zygomaticus major
Zygomaticus minor
Levator anguli oris
Buccinator
Orbicularis oris
Risorius
Mentalis
Depressor labii inferioris
Depressor anguli oris
Transversus menti

MUSCLES OF THE NECK
Superficial and lateral muscles
Platysma
Trapezius (see Upper limb)
Sternocleidomastoid

Anterior vertebral muscles
Longus colli
Longus capitis
Rectus capitis anterior
Rectus capitis lateralis

Lateral vertebral muscles
Scalenus anterior
Scalenus medius
Scalenus posterior

Suprahyoid muscles
Digastric
Stylohyoid
Mylohyoid
Geniohyoid

Infrahyoid muscles
Sternohyoid
Sternothyroid
Thyrohyoid
Omohyoid

MUSCLE GROUPS IN HEAD AND NECK

Muscles of the pharynx
Superior constrictor
Middle constrictor
Inferior constrictor
Stylopharyngeus
Palatopharyngeus
Salpingopharyngeus

Muscles of the palate
Palatoglossus
Palatopharyngeus
Tensor veli palatini
Levator veli palatini
Musculus uvulae

Muscles of the larynx
Cricothyroid
Posterior crico-arytenoid
Lateral crico-arytenoid
Transverse arytenoid
Oblique arytenoid
Aryepiglottic
Thyro-arytenoid and vocalis
Thyro-epiglottic
(Superior thyro-arytenoid)

Muscles of the tongue
Extrinsic
    Genioglossus
    Hyoglossus and chondroglossus
    Styloglossus
    Palatoglossus
Intrinsic
    Superior longitudinal
    Inferior longitudinal
    Transverse
    Vertical

Muscles of the orbit
Levator palpebrae superioris
Orbitalis
Muscles of the eyeball
    Superior rectus
    Inferior rectus
    Medial rectus
    Lateral rectus
    Superior oblique
    Inferior oblique

MUSCLES OF THE TRUNK

Suboccipital muscles
Rectus capitis posterior major
Rectus capitis posterior minor
Obliquus capitis inferior
Obliquus capitis superior

Deep muscles of the back
Splenius capitis
Splenius cervicis
Erector spinae
    Iliocostalis cervicis
    Iliocostalis thoracis
    Iliocostalis lumborum
    Longissimus capitis
    Longissimus cervicis
    Longissimus thoracis
    Spinalis capitis
    Spinalis cervicis
    Spinalis thoracis
Transversospinalis
    Semispinalis capitis
    Semispinalis cervicis
    Semispinalis thoracis
    Multifidus
    Rotatores
Interspinal
Intertransverse

MUSCLES OF THE UPPER LIMB

Connecting limb and vertebral column
Trapezius
Latissimus dorsi
Levator scapulae
Rhomboid major
Rhomboid minor

Connecting limb and thoracic wall
Pectoralis major
Pectoralis minor
Subclavius
Serratus anterior

Scapular muscles
Deltoid
Subscapularis
Supraspinatus
Infraspinatus
Teres minor
Teres major

Nerves

CRANIAL NERVES AND BRANCHES

I Olfactory (from olfactory mucous membrane)

II Optic (from retina)

III Oculomotor
  Superior branch (to superior rectus and levator
    palpebrae superioris)
  Inferior branch (to medial rectus, inferior rectus and
    inferior oblique)
    Oculomotor root to ciliary ganglion

IV Trochlear (to superior oblique)

V Trigeminal
  Sensory root
    Trigeminal ganglion
  Motor root (joining mandibular nerve)
  Ophthalmic
    Tentorial
    Lacrimal
      Communicating branch with zygomatic
    Frontal
      Supra-orbital
      Supratrochlear
    Nasociliary → anterior ethmoidal → external nasal
      Communicating branch with ciliary ganglion
      Long ciliary
      Posterior ethmoidal
      Anterior ethmoidal
        Lateral and medial internal nasal
        External nasal
      Infratrochlear
      Palpebral
  Maxillary → infra-orbital
    Meningeal
    Ganglionic branches to pterygopalatine ganglion
      Orbital
      Nasal (lateral and medial posterior superior nasal
        and nasopalatine)
      Pharyngeal
      Greater palatine
        Posterior inferior nasal
      Lesser palatine
    Zygomatic
      Zygomaticotemporal
      Zygomaticofacial
    Infra-orbital
      Superior alveolar
        Posterior, middle and anterior superior alveolar
          Superior dental plexus
            Superior dental
            Superior gingival
      Inferior palpebral
      External nasal
      Internal nasal
      Superior labial
  Mandibular *see next column*

Mandibular
  Meningeal
  Masseteric
  Deep temporal
  Nerve to lateral pterygoid
  Nerve to medial pterygoid
    Nerve to tensor veli palatini and tensor tympani
      via otic ganglion
  Buccal
  Auriculotemporal
    Nerve to external acoustic meatus
    Tympanic membrane
    Communicating branches with facial nerve
    Anterior auricular
    Superficial temporal
  Lingual
    Faucial
    Communicating branches with hypoglossal nerve
    Communicating branch with chorda tympani
    Sublingual
    Lingual
    Ganglionic branches to submandibular ganglion
  Inferior alveolar
    Mylohyoid
    Inferior dental plexus
      Inferior dental
      Inferior gingival
    Mental
      Mental
      Inferior labial

VI Abducent (to lateral rectus)

VII Facial
  Greater petrosal
  Nerve to stapedius
  Chorda tympani
  Communicating branch with tympanic plexus
  Communicating branch with vagus nerve
  Posterior auricular
    Occipital (to occipital belly of occipitofrontalis)
    Auricular (to auricular muscles)
    To digastric (posterior belly)
    To stylohyoid
    Communicating branch with glossopharyngeal nerve
  Parotid plexus

Temporal	to frontal belly of
Zygomatic	occipitofrontalis,
Buccal	muscles of facial
Marginal mandibular	expression and
Cervical	platysma

VIII Vestibulocochlear
 Cochlear (from coils of cochlea)
 Vestibular (from utricle, saccule and ampullae of
  semicircular canals)

IX Glossopharyngeal
 Tympanic
  Tubal
  Caroticotympanic
  Lesser petrosal
 Carotid sinus
 Pharyngeal
 Muscular (to stylopharyngeus)
 Tonsillar
 Lingual

X Vagus
 Meningeal
 Auricular
 Pharyngeal (to muscles of pharynx and soft palate
  except stylopharyngeus and tensor veli palatini)
 Superior cervical cardiac
 Carotid body
 Superior laryngeal
  Internal laryngeal
  External laryngeal (to cricothyroid)
 Inferior cervical cardiac
 Recurrent laryngeal
  Tracheal
  Oesophageal
  Inferior laryngeal (to muscles of larynx except
   cricothyroid)
 Thoracic cardiac
 Bronchial
 Oesophageal plexus
 Anterior vagal trunk
  Gastric
  Hepatic
 Posterior vagal trunk
  Coeliac
  Gastric

XI Accessory
 Trunk of accessory
  Internal ramus (cranial or vagal part, from cranial
   roots, to muscles of palate, except tensor veli
   palatini, and larynx via fibres joining vagus nerve)
  External ramus (spinal part, from cervical roots,
   to sternocleidomastoid and trapezius)

XII Hypoglossal
 Lingual (to muscles of tongue except palatoglossus)
 Muscular (derived from cervical nerves and including
  upper root of ansa cervicalis, to geniohyoid,
  thyrohyoid, sternohyoid, sternothyroid and
  superior belly of omohyoid)

SOME HEAD AND NECK NERVE SUPPLIES

All the muscles of	Supplied by	Except	Supplied by
Pharynx	Pharyngeal plexus	Stylo-pharyngeus	Glosso-pharyngeal nerve
Palate	Pharyngeal plexus	Tensor veli palatini	Nerve to medial pterygoid
Larynx	Recurrent laryngeal nerve	Crico-thyroid	External laryngeal nerve
Tongue	Hypoglossal nerve	Palato-glossus	Pharyngeal plexus
Facial expression (including buccinator)	Facial nerve		
Mastication	Mandibular nerve		

Nerves

CERVICAL PLEXUS AND BRANCHES

Lesser occipital C2
Great auricular C2, 3
Transverse cervical C2, 3
Supraclavicular C3, 4
Phrenic (to diaphragm) C3, 4, 5
Communicating (with vagus and hypoglossal nerves and superior cervical sympathetic ganglion)
Muscular (to rectus capitis lateralis, rectus capitis anterior, longus capitis and longus colli, and by lower root of ansa cervicalis to sternohyoid, sternothyroid and inferior belly of omohyoid) C1, 2, 3

BRACHIAL PLEXUS AND BRANCHES

Supraclavicular branches
From the roots
    To scalenes and longus colli C5, 6, 7, 8
    To join phrenic nerve C5
    Dorsal scapular (to rhomboids) C5
    Long thoracic (to serratus anterior) C5, 6, 7
From the upper trunk
    Nerve to subclavius C5, 6
    Suprascapular (to supraspinatus and infraspinatus) C5, 6

Infraclavicular branches
From the lateral cord
    Lateral pectoral (to pectoralis major and minor) C5, 6, 7
    Musculocutaneous C5, 6, 7
    Lateral root of the median C(5), 6, 7
From the medial cord
    Medial pectoral (to pectoralis major and minor) C8, T1
    Medial root of the median C8, T1
    Medial cutaneous of arm C8, T1
    Medial cutaneous of forearm C8, T1
    Ulnar C(7), 8, T1
From the posterior cord
    Upper subscapular (to subscapularis) C5, 6
    Thoracodorsal (to latissimus dorsi) C6, 7, 8
    Lower subscapular (to subscapularis and teres major) C5, 6
    Axillary C5, 6
    Radial C5, 6, 7, 8, T1

Lymphatic System

THORACIC DUCT AND RIGHT LYMPHATIC DUCT

Thoracic duct
Left jugular trunk
Left subclavian trunk
Left bronchomediastinal trunk

Right lymphatic duct
Right jugular trunk
Right subclavian trunk
Right bronchomediastinal trunk

Cisterna chyli
Left lumbar trunk
Right lumbar trunk
Intestinal trunks

LYMPH NODES OF THE HEAD AND NECK

Deep cervical
Superior (including jugulodigastric)
Inferior (including jugulo-omohyoid)

Draining superficial tissues in the head
Occipital
Retro-auricular (mastoid)
Parotid
Buccal (facial)

Draining superficial tissues in the neck
Submandibular
Submental
Anterior cervical
Superficial cervical

Draining deep tissues in the neck
Retropharyngeal
Paratracheal
Lingual
Infrahyoid
Prelaryngeal
Pretracheal

Arteries

AORTA AND BRANCHES

Ascending aorta → arch of aorta → thoracic aorta → abdominal aorta

Ascending aorta
Right coronary
  Marginal
  Posterior interventricular
Left coronary
  Circumflex
  Anterior interventricular

Arch of aorta
Brachiocephalic trunk
  Right common carotid
    Right internal carotid
    Right external carotid
  Right subclavian → axillary → brachial
  Thyroidea ima (occasional)
Left common carotid
  Left internal carotid
  Left external carotid
Left subclavian → axillary → brachial

SUBCLAVIAN ARTERY AND BRANCHES

Subclavian → axillary → brachial
  Vertebral
    Prevertebral part
    Transversarial (cervical) part
      Spinal (radicular)
      Muscular
    Atlantic part
    Intracranial part
      Anterior and posterior meningeal
      Anterior spinal
      Posterior inferior cerebellar
        Choroidal of fourth ventricle
        To cerebellar tonsil
        Medial and lateral medullary
        Posterior spinal
  Basilar (from union of both vertebrals)
    Anterior inferior cerebellar
    Labyrinthine
    Pontine
    Mesencephalic
    Superior cerebellar
    Posterior cerebral
      Precommunicating part
        Posteromedial central
      Postcommunicating part
        Posterolateral central
        Thalamic
        Medial and lateral posterior choroidal
        Peduncular
      Terminal (cortical) part
        Lateral occipital
          Anterior, middle and posterior temporal
        Medial occipital
          Dorsal corpus callosal
          Parietal
          Calcarine
          Occipitotemporal
  Thyrocervical trunk
    Inferior thyroid
      Inferior laryngeal
      Glandular
      Pharyngeal
      Oesophageal
      Tracheal
      Ascending cervical
        Spinal
    Superficial cervical
    Suprascapular
      Acromial
  Internal thoracic
  Costocervical trunk
    Deep cervical
    Superior intercostal
      First posterior intercostal
      Second posterior intercostal
        Dorsal
        Spinal
  Dorsal scapular

CAROTID ARTERIES AND BRANCHES

Internal carotid

Cervical part
  Carotid sinus
Petrous part
  Caroticotympanic
  Pterygoid canal
Cavernous part
  Basal and marginal tentorial
  Meningeal
  To trigeminal ganglion
  Trigeminal and trochlear
  Cavernous sinus
  Inferior hypophysial
Cerebral part
  Superior hypophysial
  Ophthalmic
    Central of retina
    Lacrimal
      Anastomotic branch with middle meningeal
      Lateral palpebral
    Short and long posterior ciliary
    Muscular
      Anterior ciliary
    Anterior and posterior conjunctival
    Episcleral
    Supra-orbital
    Posterior ethmoidal
    Anterior ethmoidal
      Anterior meningeal
    Medial palpebral
    Supratrochlear
    Dorsal nasal
  Anterior cerebral
    Precommunicating part
      Anteromedial central (thalamostriate)
      Short central
      Long central (recurrent)
      Anterior communicating
    Postcommunicating part (pericallosal)
      Medial frontobasal (orbitofrontal)
      Callosomarginal
        Anteromedial frontal
        Intermediomedial frontal
        Posteromedial frontal
        Cingular
      Paracentral
      Precuneal
      Parieto-occipital
  Middle cerebral *see next column*

Middle cerebral
  Sphenoidal part
    Anterolateral central (thalamostriate)
      Medial and lateral (striate)
  Insular part
    Insular
    Lateral frontobasal (orbitofrontal)
    Anterior, intermediate and posterior temporal
  Terminal (cortical) part
    To central sulcus
    To precentral sulcus
    To postcentral sulcus
    Anterior and posterior parietal
    To angular gyrus
Anterior choroidal
  Choroidal of lateral ventricle
  Choroidal of third ventricle
  To anterior perforated substance
  To optic tract
  To lateral geniculate body
  To internal capsule
  To globus pallidus
  To tail of caudate nucleus
  To tuber cinereum
  To hypothalamic nuclei
  To substantia nigra
  To red nucleus
  To amygdaloid body
Posterior communicating (joining posterior cerebral)
  Chiasmatic
  To oculomotor nerve
  Thalamic
  Hypothalamic
  To tail of caudate nucleus

External carotid
Superior thyroid
  Infrahyoid
  Sternocleidomastoid
  Superior laryngeal
  Cricothyroid
Ascending pharyngeal
  Posterior meningeal
  Pharyngeal
  Inferior tympanic
Lingual
  Suprahyoid
  Sublingual
  Dorsal lingual
  Deep lingual
Facial
  Ascending palatine
  Tonsillar
  Submental
  Glandular
  Inferior labial
  Superior labial
  Angular
Occipital
  Mastoid
  Auricular
  Sternocleidomastoid
  Meningeal
  Occipital
  Descending
Posterior auricular
  Stylomastoid
  Posterior tympanic
    Mastoid
    Stapedial
  Auricular
  Occipital
Superficial temporal
  Parotid
  Transverse facial
  Anterior auricular
  Zygomatico-orbital
  Middle temporal
  Frontal
  Parietal
Maxillary *see next column*

Maxillary
  Deep auricular
  Anterior tympanic
  Inferior alveolar
    Dental
    Mylohyoid
    Mental
  Middle meningeal
    Accessory meningeal
    Petrosal
    Superior tympanic
    Frontal
    Parietal
    Orbital
    Anastomotic branch with lacrimal
  Masseteric
  Deep temporal
  Pterygoid
  Buccal
  Posterior superior alveolar
    Dental
  Infra-orbital
    Anterior superior alveolar
      Dental
  Pterygoid canal
  Descending palatine
    Greater palatine
    Lesser palatine
  Sphenopalatine
    Posterior, lateral and septal nasal

Veins

TRIBUTARIES OF MAJOR VEINS
Superior vena cava
Left brachiocephalic
  Left internal jugular
  Left subclavian
  Left vertebral
  Left supreme (first posterior) intercostal
  Left superior intercostal (2–4)
  Inferior thyroid
  Thymic
  Pericardial
Right brachiocephalic
  Right internal jugular
  Right subclavian
  Right vertebral
  Right supreme (first posterior) intercostal
Azygos

Internal jugular
Inferior petrosal sinus
Pharyngeal
Lingual
Facial
Superior thyroid
Middle thyroid

External jugular
Posterior auricular
Posterior branch of retromandibular
Occipital
Posterior external jugular
Suprascapular
Transverse of neck
Anterior jugular

Retromandibular
Superficial temporal
Maxillary
Transverse facial
Pterygoid plexus
  Middle meningeal
  Greater palatine
  Sphenopalatine
  Buccal
  Dental
  Deep facial
  Inferior ophthalmic
Anterior branch to join facial
Posterior branch to external jugular

Facial
Supratrochlear
Supra-orbital
Superior ophthalmic
Palpebral
External nasal
Labial
Deep facial
Submental
Submandibular
Tonsillar
External palatine (paratonsillar)

DURAL VENOUS SINUSES
Posterosuperior group
Superior sagittal
Inferior sagittal
Straight
Transverse
Sigmoid
Petrosquamous
Occipital

Antero-inferior group
Cavernous
Intercavernous
Inferior petrosal
Superior petrosal
Sphenoparietal
Basilar
Middle meningeal veins

EMISSARY VEINS
The most common are found in the
Parietal foramen
Mastoid foramen
Foramen lacerum
Foramen ovale
Venous (emissary sphenoidal) foramen
Carotid canal
Hypoglossal canal
Condylar canal

CEREBRAL VEINS
Superficial cerebral veins
  Superior cerebral
  Superficial middle cerebral
    Superior anastomotic
    Inferior anastomotic
  Inferior cerebral
Deep cerebral veins
  Great cerebral
    Internal cerebral
      Thalamostriate
      Choroidal
    Basal
      Anterior cerebral
      Deep middle cerebral
      Striate

Skull Foramina

INSIDE THE SKULL

MIDDLE CRANIAL FOSSA

Optic canal: in the sphenoid between the body and the two roots of the lesser wing
Optic nerve
Ophthalmic artery

Superior orbital fissure: in the sphenoid between the body and the greater and lesser wings, with a fragment of the frontal bone at the lateral extremity
Oculomotor, trochlear and abducent nerves
Lacrimal, frontal and nasociliary nerves
Filaments from the internal carotid (sympathetic) plexus
Orbital branch of the middle meningeal artery
Recurrent branch of the lacrimal artery
Superior ophthalmic vein

Foramen rotundum: in the greater wing of the sphenoid
Maxillary nerve

Foramen ovale: in the greater wing of the sphenoid
Mandibular nerve
Lesser petrosal nerve (usually)
Accessory meningeal artery
Emissary veins (from cavernous sinus to pterygoid plexus)

Foramen spinosum: in the greater wing of the sphenoid
Middle meningeal vessels
Meningeal branch of the mandibular nerve

Venous (emissary sphenoidal) foramen: in 40% of skulls, in the greater wing of the sphenoid medial to the foramen ovale
Emissary vein (from the cavernous sinus to the pterygoid plexus)

Petrosal (innominate) foramen: occasional, in the greater wing of the sphenoid, medial to the foramen spinosum
Lesser petrosal nerve (if not through foramen ovale)

Foramen lacerum: between the sphenoid, apex of the petrous temporal and the basilar part of the occipital
Internal carotid artery (entering from behind and emerging above)
Greater petrosal nerve (entering from above and behind, and leaving anteriorly as nerve of pterygoid canal)
Nerve of pterygoid canal (leaving through anterior wall)
A meningeal branch of the ascending pharyngeal artery
Emissary veins (from the cavernous sinus to the pterygoid plexus)

Hiatus for the greater petrosal nerve: in the tegmen tympani of the petrous temporal, in front of the arcuate eminence
Greater petrosal nerve
Petrosal branch of the middle meningeal artery

Hiatus for the lesser petrosal nerve: in the tegmen tympani of the petrous temporal, about 3 mm in front of the hiatus for the greater petrosal nerve
Lesser petrosal nerve

ANTERIOR CRANIAL FOSSA

Foramina in the cribriform plate of the ethmoid
Olfactory nerve filaments
Anterior ethmoidal nerve and vessels

Foramen caecum: between the frontal crest of the frontal bone and the ethmoid in front of the crista galli
Emissary vein (between nose and superior sagittal sinus)

POSTERIOR CRANIAL FOSSA

Internal acoustic meatus: in the posterior surface of the petrous temporal
Facial nerve
Vestibulocochlear nerve
Labyrinthine artery

Aqueduct of the vestibule: in the petrous temporal about 1 cm behind the internal acoustic meatus
Endolymphatic duct and sac
A branch from the meningeal branch of the occipital artery
A vein (from the labyrinth and vestibule to the sigmoid sinus)

Jugular foramen: between the jugular fossa of the petrous temporal and the occipital bone
Glossopharyngeal, vagus and accessory nerves
Meningeal branches of the vagus nerve
Inferior petrosal sinus
Internal jugular vein
A meningeal branch of the occipital artery

Hypoglossal canal: in the occipital bone above the anterior part of the condyle
Hypoglossal nerve and its (recurrent) meningeal branch
A meningeal branch of the ascending pharyngeal artery
Emissary vein (from the basilar plexus to the internal jugular vein)

Condylar canal: occasional, from the lower part of the sigmoid groove in the lateral part of the occipital bone to the condylar fossa on the external surface of the occipital bone behind the condyle
Emissary vein (from the sigmoid sinus to occipital veins)
A meningeal branch of the occipital artery

Mastoid foramen: in the petrous temporal near the posterior margin of the lower part of the sigmoid groove, passing backwards to open behind the mastoid process
Emissary vein (from the sigmoid sinus to occipital veins)
A meningeal branch of the occipital artery

Foramen magnum: in the occipital bone
Apical ligament of the odontoid process of the axis
Tectorial membrane
Medulla oblongata and meninges (including first digitations of denticulate ligament)
Spinal parts of the accessory nerves
Meningeal branches of upper cervical nerves
Vertebral arteries
Anterior spinal artery
Posterior spinal arteries

Skull Foramina

IN THE BASE OF THE SKULL EXTERNALLY

Foramen lacerum
Foramen ovale
Foramen spinosum
Jugular foramen   } see INSIDE THE SKULL
Hypoglossal canal
Condylar canal
Mastoid foramen
Foramen magnum

Inferior orbital fissure – see IN THE ORBIT

Lateral incisive foramen: opens into the incisive fossa, in the midline at the front of the hard palate
Nasopalatine nerve
Greater palatine vessels

Greater palatine foramen: between the maxilla and the palatine bone at the lateral border of the hard palate behind the palatomaxillary fissure
Greater palatine nerve and vessels

Lesser palatine foramina: two or three, in the inferior and medial aspects of the pyramidal process of the palatine bone
Lesser palatine nerves and vessels

Palatovaginal canal: between lower surface of the vaginal process of the root of the medial pterygoid plate and the upper surface of the sphenoidal process of the palatine bone
Pharyngeal branch of the pterygopalatine ganglion
Pharyngeal branch of the maxillary artery

Vomerovaginal canal: occasional, medial to the palatovaginal canal, between the upper surface of the vaginal process of the root of the medial pterygoid plate and the lower surface of the ala of the vomer
Pharyngeal branch of the sphenopalatine artery

Petrosquamous fissure: between the squamous temporal and the tegmen tympani
Petrosquamous vein

Petrotympanic fissure: between the tympanic part of the temporal bone and the tegmen tympani
Chorda tympani
Anterior ligament of the malleus
Anterior tympanic branch of the maxillary artery

Cochlear canaliculus: in the petrous temporal, at the apex of a notch in front of the medial part of the jugular fossa
Perilymphatic duct
Emissary vein (from the cochlea to the internal jugular vein or inferior petrosal sinus)

Carotid canal: in the inferior surface of the petrous temporal
Internal carotid artery
Internal carotid (sympathetic) plexus
Internal carotid venous plexus (from the cavernous sinus to the internal jugular vein)

Tympanic canaliculus: in the inferior surface of the petrous temporal, on the ridge of bone between the carotid canal and the jugular fossa
Tympanic branch of the glossopharyngeal nerve
Inferior tympanic branch of the ascending pharyngeal artery

Mastoid canaliculus: in the inferior surface of the petrous temporal, on the lateral wall of the jugular fossa
Auricular branch of the vagus nerve

Stylomastoid foramen: between the styloid and mastoid processes of the temporal bone
Facial nerve
Stylomastoid branch of the posterior auricular artery

IN THE ORBIT

Superior orbital fissure
Optic canal } see INSIDE THE SKULL

Frontal notch or foramen: in the supra-orbital margin of the frontal bone one fingerbreadth from the midline
Supratrochlear nerve and vessels

Supra-orbital notch or foramen: in the supra-orbital margin of the frontal bone two fingerbreadths from the midline
Supra-orbital nerve and vessels

Anterior ethmoidal foramen: in the medial wall of the orbit between the orbital part of the frontal bone and the ethmoid labyrinth
Anterior ethmoidal nerve and vessels

Posterior ethmoidal foramen: occasional, 1–2 cm behind the anterior ethmoidal foramen
Posterior ethmoidal nerve and vessels

Zygomatico-orbital foramen: in the orbital surface of the zygomatic bone
Zygomatic branch of the maxillary nerve

Nasolacrimal canal: at the front, lower, medial corner of the orbit formed by the lacrimal bone and maxilla
Nasolacrimal duct

Inferior orbital fissure: towards the back of the orbit, between the maxilla and the greater wing of the sphenoid
Maxillary nerve
Zygomatic nerve
Orbital branches of the pterygopalatine ganglion
Infra-orbital vessels
Inferior ophthalmic veins

Infra-orbital canal: in the orbital surface of the maxilla
Infra-orbital nerve and vessels

MISCELLANEOUS

Infra-orbital foramen: the anterior opening of the infra-orbital canal, in the maxilla below the infra-orbital margin
Infra-orbital nerve and vessels

Mental foramen: on the outer surface of the body of the mandible below the second premolar tooth or slightly more anteriorly
Mental nerve and vessels

Mandibular foramen: on the inner surface of the ramus of the mandible, overlapped anteriorly and medially by the lingula
Inferior alveolar nerve and vessels

Foramina in the infratemporal (posterior) surface of the maxilla
Posterior superior alveolar nerves and vessels

Pterygomaxillary fissure: between the lateral pterygoid plate and the infratemporal (posterior) surface of the maxilla, and continuous above with the posterior end of the inferior orbital fissure
Maxillary artery (entering pterygopalatine fossa)
Maxillary nerve (entering inferior orbital fissure)
Sphenopalatine veins

Sphenopalatine foramen: at the upper end of the perpendicular plate of the palatine between its orbital and sphenoidal processes and (above) the body of the sphenoid; in the medial wall of the pterygopalatine fossa (viewed laterally through the pterygomaxillary fissure) and lateral wall of the nasal cavity (viewed medially)
Nasopalatine and posterior superior nasal nerves
Sphenopalatine vessels

Foramina in the perpendicular plate of the palatine
Posterior inferior nasal nerves

Pterygoid canal: at the root of the pterygoid process of the sphenoid in line with the medial pterygoid plate, leading from the anterior wall of the foramen lacerum to the posterior wall of the pterygopalatine fossa (and only clearly seen in a disarticulated sphenoid)
Nerve of the pterygoid canal
Artery of the pterygoid canal

Musculotubular canal: at the lateral side of the apex of the petrous temporal, at the junction of the petrous and squamous parts, and divided by a bony septum into upper and lower semicanals
Tensor tympani (upper semicanal)
Auditory tube (lower semicanal)

Parietal foramen: in the parietal bone near the posterosuperior (occipital) angle
Emissary vein (from the superior sagittal sinus to the scalp)

Index